**Volume 02
Issue 03
November 2007**

The Senses & Society

⊛BERG

AIMS AND SCOPE

A heightened interest in the role of the senses in culture and society is sweeping the human sciences, supplanting older paradigms and challenging conventional theories of representation.

This pioneering journal provides a crucial forum for the exploration of this vital new area of inquiry. It brings together groundbreaking work in the humanities and social sciences and incorporates cutting-edge developments in art, design, and architecture. Every volume contains something for and about each of the senses, both singly and in all sorts of novel configurations.

Sensation is fundamental to our experience of the world. Shaped by culture, gender, and class, the senses mediate between mind and body, idea and object, self and environment. The senses are increasingly extended beyond the body through technology, and catered to by designers and marketers, yet persistently elude all efforts to capture and control them. Artists now experiment with the senses in bold new ways, disrupting conventional canons of aesthetics.

- How is perception shaped by cultures and technologies?
- In what ways are the senses sites for the production and practice of ideologies of gender, class, and race?
- How many senses are there to "aesthetics"?
- What are the social implications of the increasing commercialization of sensation?
- How might a focus on the cultural life of the senses yield new insights into processes of cognition and emotion?

The Senses & Society aims to:

- Explore the intersection between culture and the senses
- Promote research on the politics of perception and the aesthetics of everyday life
- Address architectural, marketing, and design initiatives in relation to the senses
- Publish reviews of books and multi-sensory exhibitions throughout the world
- Publish special issues concentrating on particular themes relating to the senses

To submit an article, please write to Michael Bull at:

The Senses and Society
Department of Media & Film Studies
University of Sussex
Brighton
Sussex
BN1 9QQ
UK

email:
senses@sussex.ac.uk or
m.bull@sussex.ac.uk

Books for review should be sent to David Howes at:

The Senses and Society
Department of Sociology and Anthropology
Concordia University
1455 de Maisonneuve Boulevard West
Montreal, Quebec
H3G 1M8
CANADA

email:
senses@alcor.concordia.ca
howesd@alcor.concordia.ca

Comments and suggestions regarding Sensory Design reviews should be addressed to Joy Monice Malnar

email:
malnar@uiuc.edu

Comments and suggestions regarding multisensory exhibition and conference reviews should be addressed to Jim Drobnick

email:
jdrobnick@faculty.ocad.ca

©2007 Berg. All rights reserved.
No part of this publication may be reproduced or utilized in any form or by any means, electronic or mechanical, including photocopying and recording, or by any information storage or retrieval system, without permission in writing from the publisher.

ISSN (print): 1745-8927
ISSN (online): 1745-8935

The Senses and Society is indexed by:
AIO – Anthropological Index Online (Royal Anthropological Library); CSA: Sociological Abstracts; Baywood's Abstracts in Anthropology; CSA: ARTbibliographies Modern; CSA: British Humanities Index; and CSA: DAAI – Design and Applied Arts Index

Berg Publishers is a member of CrossRef

SUBSCRIPTION INFORMATION

Three issues per volume.
One volume per annum.
2007: Volume 2

ONLINE
www.bergpublishers.com

BY MAIL
Berg Publishers
C/o Customer Services
Turpin Distribution
Pegasus Drive
Stratton Business Park
Biggleswade
Bedfordshire SG18 8TQ
UK

BY FAX
+44 (0)1767 601640

BY TELEPHONE
+44 (0)1767 604951

BY EMAIL
custserv@turpin-distribution.com

INQUIRIES
Julia Hall, Managing Editor
email: jhall@bergpublishers.com

Production: Ian Critchley, email: icritchley@bergpublishers.com

Advertising and subscriptions:
Veruschka Selbach,
email: vselbach@bergpublishers.com

SUBSCRIPTION RATES

Print
Institutional: (1 year) $300/£165;
(2 year) $480/£264
Individual: (1 year) $70/£40*; (2 year) $112/£64*

Online only
Institutional and individual: (1 year) $240, £130; (2 year) $384, £208

*This price is available only to personal subscribers and must be prepaid by personal cheque or credit card

Free online subscription for institutional subscribers

Full color images available online

Access your electronic subscription through www.ingenta.com

REPRINTS FOR MAILING

Copies of individual articles may be obtained from the publishers at the appropriate fees.
Write to

Berg Publishers
1st Floor, Angel Court
81 St Clements Street
Oxford OX4 1AW
UK

Founding Editors
Michael Bull and David Howes

EDITORIAL BOARD

Managing Editor
Michael Bull, University of Sussex, UK

Editors
Paul Gilroy, London School of Economics, UK

David Howes, Concordia University, Canada

Douglas Kahn, University of California, Davis, USA

Sensory Design Editor
Joy Monice Malnar, University of Illinois, Urbana-Champaign

Book Reviews Editor
David Howes, Concordia University

Exhibition and Conference Reviews Editor
Jim Drobnick, Ontario College of Art and Design, Toronto, Canada

ADVISORY BOARD

Alison Clarke, *University of Vienna, Austria*

Steven Connor, *University of London, UK*

Alain Corbin, *Université de Paris I, La Sorbonne, France*

Ruth Finnegan, *Open University, UK*

Jukka Gronow, *University of Uppsala, Sweden*

Peter Charles Hoffer, *University of Georgia, USA*

Caroline Jones, *Massachusetts Institute of Technology, USA*

Barbara Kirshenblatt-Gimblett, *New York University, USA*

Margaret Morse, *University of California at Santa Cruz, USA*

Ruth Phillips, *Carleton University, Canada*

Leigh Schmidt, *Princeton University, USA*

Mark Smith, *University of South Carolina, USA*

Jonathan Sterne, *McGill University, Canada*

Paul Stoller, *West Chester University, USA*

Michael Syrotinski, *University of Aberdeen, UK*

Nigel Thrift, *University of Warwick, UK*

Fran Tonkiss, *London School of Economics, UK*

Typeset by JS Typesetting Ltd, Porthcawl, Mid Glamorgan
Printed in the UK

The Senses & Society

**Volume 02
Issue 03
November 2007**

Contents

Articles

277 **Resonant Texts: Sounds of the American Public Library**
Shannon Mattern

303 **In Search of Sound: Authenticity, Healing, and Redemption in the Early Modern State**
Penelope Gouk

329 **Fear in Paradise: The Affective Registers of the English Lake District Landscape Re-visited**
Divya P. Tolia-Kelly

353 **Surprising the Senses**
Geke D.S. Ludden, Hendrik N.J. Schifferstein and Paul Hekkert

Sensory Design

363 **Material Experience: Peter Zumthor's Thermal Bath at Vals**
Scott Murray

Book Reviews

371 **Cottage in a Boudoir: Ann Bermingham (ed.), *Sensation and Sensibility: Viewing Gainsborough's* Cottage Door**
   Reviewed by Jessica Riskin

377 **Rich Pickings: Carolyn Korsmeyer (ed.), *The Taste Culture Reader: Experiencing Food and Drink*, and Denise Gigante, *Taste: A Literary History***
   Reviewed by Jean Duruz

Exhibition and Conference Reviews

385 **Tropicália: A Revolution in Brazilian Culture**
Reviewed by Jonathan Goodman

391 **Luigi Russolo's Art of Noises**
Reviewed by James Mansell

397 **Between Art and Science**
"Making Sense of Art, Making Art of Sense"
Reviewed by Patrizia Di Bello

Resonant Texts: Sounds of the American Public Library

Shannon Mattern

Shannon Mattern is an assistant professor at The New School in New York. Her book, *The New Downtown Library: Designing With Communities*, was published by the University of Minnesota Press.
MatternS@newschool.edu

ABSTRACT   Public libraries have long been associated with silence and order. Historians have argued that the architecture of library buildings has served in disciplining patrons into silent reading subjects. I argue that, in light of evolving, subjective definitions of and responses to noise, changing philosophies of librarianship and library design and the proliferation of media formats and the sounds they emit, we need to consider new ways of thinking about sound in the library, not as something to be eliminated or controlled, but as something to be orchestrated, and even *designed for*. In order to do so, I propose that we consider first what sounds people, buildings and media make, and then use architectural design to promote their cooperative interaction.

KEYWORDS: public libraries, acoustics, noise, media reception, habitus

✚ In Salt Lake City, librarians wear buttons displaying the house rule: "No shhh!"
Libraries and noise seem to have made their peace. The new Salt Lake City Public Library, like many recently opened American public library buildings, is designed to accommodate newer, noisier kinds of work – work that involves spirited discussion between collaborators, work with media formats that make once-mute pages speak, work underscored by the clicking of laptop keys. These are the sounds of a public library that has proven its continued relevance and *resonance* in an age when new technologies and privatized services were to have spelled the institution's demise.

But not everyone is happy about the sounds emanating from the stacks. In one of the many focus groups the Seattle Public Library hosted while planning their new building in the late 1990s, some patrons requested private study carrels, cell-phone-free zones and a "laptop-free" area where they could study without sonic distraction. Sam Demas at Carleton College has logged similar requests from students. "Daydreaming, contemplation, thinking, reading, and, yes, sleeping are cherished private, even intimate, aspects of the student experience supported by the library," he writes. "Where does one go for peace and quiet?" (Demas 2005, n.p.). Not the *public* library, apparently, lamented author Sally Tisdale in a *Harper's* article. Tisdale marvels that "today's library is trendy, up-to-date, plugged in… It's a hip, fun place, the library" (1997: 66). Yet all of this excitement has compromised what she regards as one of the unique, core functions of the institution:

> The boundaries that have kept the library a refuge from the street and the marketplace are being deliberately torn down in the name of access and popularity. No one seems to believe that there is a public need for refuge; no one seems to understand that people who can't afford computers and video games can hardly afford silence (Tisdale 1997: 74).

The public library – at one time represented, fairly or not, by the bespectacled librarian perched behind a fortress-like desk, finger pressed to her lips (see Figure 1) – has, in some places, chosen a new ambassador: the roving librarian equipped with handheld device and cell phone, combing the stacks for patrons in need of assistance. And in many cities' new downtown libraries, the scene that greets people as they walk through the main entrance is not rows of patrons hunched silently over books, but, rather, a bustling cafe, high school students chatting over a magazine, or a local author giving a reading.

When these buildings are designed thoughtfully, tranquility need not give way to clamor. There is room for both acoustic conditions, and plenty in-between. Elsewhere, I discuss the designs of several new urban public library buildings, and particularly how their mix

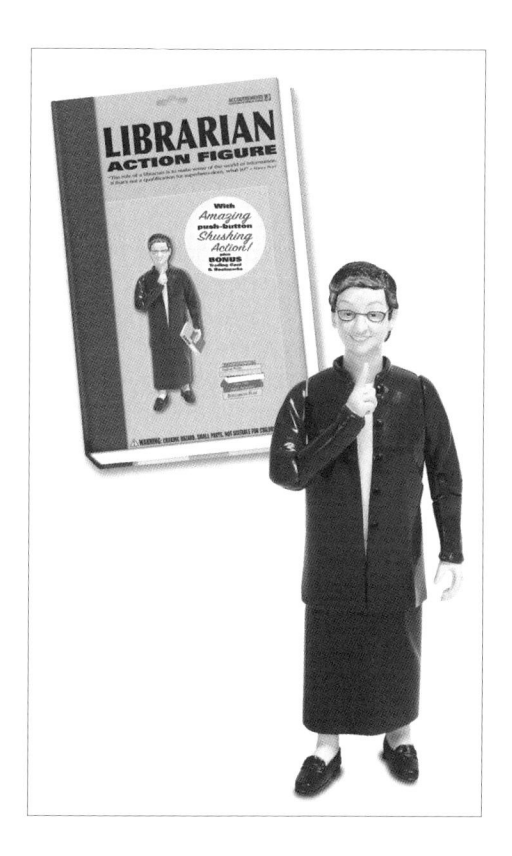

Figure 1
Nancy Pearl, Seattle public librarian and author of *Book Lust*, has had an action figure – with amazing "shushing action" – made in her likeness. Image Copyright Archie McPhee.

of media and non-media functions necessitates programmatic areas with disparate characters – visual, haptic and sonic (Mattern 2007). The sound environments in these buildings range from the surveilled silence of the special collections rooms to the vibrant cacophony of the teens' libraries to the contained commotion in private listening booths. Each of the activities that takes place in a library – including reading, viewing, media-making, even dating – has its own appropriate sound conditions. And the designers of many of these new library buildings have taken these sonic demands into consideration at various stages of the design process – from siting to choosing finishing materials. In the following pages, I will discuss the varied sound environments in American library buildings – and how these sound spaces shape relationships between people, media and architecture. My primary interest is the contemporary library, but we will examine some nineteenth and early twentieth century buildings along the way. I argue that in light of evolving, subjective definitions of and responses to noise, changing philosophies of librarianship and library design and the proliferation of media formats and the sounds they emit, we need to consider new ways of thinking about sound in the library. We need to think of it not as something to be eliminated or controlled, but as something to be orchestrated, and even *designed for*. In order to do so, In order to do so, I propose that we consider first what sounds people, buildings, and media make, and then use architectural design to promote their cooperative interaction.

Sound Studies

This paper fits into the growing field of "sound studies," which, according to broadcasting historian Michelle Hilmes, has become, through the work of scholars and practitioners in various disciplines, less "the study of sound itself, or as practices of aurality within a particular industry or field, than of the cultural contexts out of which sound media emerged and which they in turn work to create: *sound culture*" (2005: 249). Of particular note – and the focus of Hilmes' 2005 book review in *American Quarterly* – are Jonathan Sterne's (2003) *The Audible Past: Cultural Origins of Sound Reproduction* and Emily Thompson's (2002) *The Soundscape of Modernity: Architectural Acoustics and the Culture of Listening in America, 1900 to 1930*. Sterne examines the development of a set of practices of listening – an "audile technique" – that was specifically modern, "articulated to science, reason, [and] instrumentality" (2003: 23). While Sterne focuses on such modern instruments and machines as the phonautograph, the stethoscope and the telegraph, Thompson addresses other realms of modern technique: architectural design and the nascent field of acoustic engineering. She links modern listening practices to modern techniques for producing space. Sterne does not ignore the spatial qualities of sound – he does address the privatization and cellularization of listening spaces – but Hilmes singles out Thompson's book for "its attention to the physical environment in which listening takes place" (Hilmes 2005: 255). Thompson joins others – including a host of philosophers, musicians and architects – who have examined the relationships between architecture and hearing – or, more generally, between space and sound.

Thompson's survey encompasses architectural types ranging from concert halls to churches to office buildings, but does not extend to libraries. Historian Ari Kelman fills this gap with "The Sound of the Civic: Reading Noise at the New York Public Library"(2001). Kelman examines how the library – the 42nd Street Humanities and Social Sciences Library, specifically – functions as a "social space" that produces the disciplined, *silent* reading subjects essential for social order and civil society. "By staging, scripting, and silencing encounters between people and people, and between people and texts, the ... Library becomes powerful and deeply productive of a civic, if eternally noisy city," he writes (25). Kelman places "noise" – the urban noise outside the library, the internal noise inimical to concentrated study, the noise of the Foucauldian "disciplinary machine" – at the center of his inquiry, yet he sometimes conflates environmental and incidental noises with "noise" as it is defined in the "transmission model" of communication theory – that is, interference between sender and receiver. He even occasionally equates "noise" with "disagreement," which may result from, but need not always be the consequence of, interference in communication. We are unsure of how the noise of the institution-as-"disciplinary machine" either drowns out or harmonizes with the noises of library media and human presence. In regard to the latter, conversation is clearly discouraged in this space, yet other sonic traces of human presence – "people walking, writing, typing" – he says, "are all involved in the performance and the production of the civic... These audial eruptions are not considered noise in the library because they are expected and even necessary for the machine to function" (38).

Composer R. Murray Schafer acknowledges that noise can mean either (1) unwanted sound, (2) unmusical sound, (3) any loud sound or (4) disturbance in any signaling system (1977: 183). Kelman uses "noise" in accordance with both Schafer's first and fourth definitions, while most librarians and acoustical designers use noise to refer to "unwanted sound," which may *include* loud sounds (3) and those that interrupt any interpersonal or mediated communication (4). Drawing on anthropologist Mary Douglas's definition of dirt as "matter out of place," historian Peter Bailey proposes that noise refers to "sound out of place" (1996: 50). Fellow historian Karin Bijsterveld identifies qualities of sounds that characterize them as negative or positive, as "noise" or not:

> "unwanted sound"... has often been associated with a terrifying disruption of a specific social order, whereas rhythmic and/or loud, positively evaluated sounds have been associated with strength, power, significance, masculinity, progress, prosperity and, last but not least, *control* (2001: 42).

Philosopher Theodor Lessing agrees, according to Lawrence Baron (1982), that making noise is a "sublimated manifestation of the 'will to power'" (167). Noise, by blaring in opposition to sometimes faceless social forces, can be an "expressive and communicative resource that registers collective and individual identities, including those of [gender, class] nation, race, and ethnicity," Bailey explains (1996:64).

But if noise renders power, expresses identity and exerts control, its opposite – *silence* – can often do the same. Again, Bailey: "Silence, we might say, is the sound of authority – generational, patriarchal and formidably inscribed in the regimes of church and state" (1996: 53). Both *enforced silence* and *freedom from noise* represent forms of power.

It is clear that neither the distinction between nor the meanings of noise and silence are fixed or universally understood. "Noise and silence refer to deeply-rooted cultural hierarchies," Bijsterveld (2001) acknowledges. These historically and culturally determined distinctions also depend, as Bailey reminds us, on the position of hearing and sound "in the sense ratio of any particular era or culture" (1996: 55). Cultural historian Hillel Schwartz concludes that noise is less an issue "of tone or decibel than of social temperament, class background, and cultural desire, all historically conditioned" (2004: 52).

The overdetermined and subjective characterization of "noise" has been made abundantly clear by the campaigns designed to define and control it – particularly the noise abatement campaigns of the early twentieth century. Because these campaigns are addressed elsewhere, I will not discuss them here.[1] However, it is worth noting the similarities between noise abatement and public library supporters in their motivation and tactics. Raymond Smilor, a pioneer in the study of noise politics, argues that noise "gave people the opportunity to express their anxiety over machine technology, [and] to test their ability to control their physical surroundings"; noise provided a seemingly concrete enemy in their fight against industrialization's "disruption of a [preexisting] social order," to borrow Bijsterveld's phrase (Smilor 1977: 36). Debates over library policies and designs provided a similarly concrete, seemingly "manageable" means for dealing with large, abstract social shifts, like urbanization and immigration – and both the anti-noise and library movements advocated for similar strategies, like effective space planning. Although "noise," specifically, was not central to the library supporters' agendas, what it represented – disorder, inefficiency, incivility – was precisely what the library was designed to combat, say many library historians. And as we turn now to examine the history of sound in the library, we should keep in mind what the "din" reformers learned about their enemy: that "noise" often resists a totalizing definition and finds a way to leak through physical and regulatory barriers.

Progressivism, Noise and the Public Library
Has library propriety always called for silence? Remembering St. Augustine and Ambrose, Alberto Manguel, in *A History of Reading* (1996), wonders,

> Was it different then, in the days of Athens or Pergamum, trying to concentrate with dozens of readers laying out tables or unfurling scrolls, mumbling away to themselves an infinity of different scores? Perhaps they didn't hear the din; perhaps they didn't know that it was possible to read in any other way. In any case, we have no recorded instances of readers complaining of the noise in Greek or Roman libraries (44).

If the sounds of reading were not bothersome, perhaps we cannot call them *noise*. We receive a different account from Claude Héméré, Librarian of the Sorbonne (1638–43), who describes appropriate behavior in his library:

Resonant Texts: Sounds of the American Public Library

> A reader who sat down in the space between two desks, as they rose to a height of five feet … neither saw nor disturbed any one else who might be reading or writing in another place by talking or by any other interruption, unless the other student wished it, or paid attention to any question that might be put to him. It was required, by the ancient rules of the library, that reading, writing, and handling of books should go forward in complete silence (quoted in Clark 1894: 40).

Historian Donald Oehlerts describes the Library Company in Philadelphia, which moved in 1790 into a new building, as the "earliest example in the United States of the use of the second floor for reading rooms to obtain better lighting, more space, and less noise and dust from the street" (1991: 4).

Héméré and Oehlerts touch on a theme that is central to Thompson's argument: that the organization of space can be used for sound (and social) control. The placement of the library within the town or city not only reflected the place of culture in the community, but also suggested what type of a sonic environment the library was to be. Late-nineteenth- and early twentieth-century library trustees, inspired by City Beautiful planning principles, often placed their large central libraries in not-so-central locations, clustered with other cultural institutions in a park-like setting and removed from the downtown business district and its potentially "sullying" – and noisy – influences (Van Slyck 1995: 82).

The siting of these late-nineteenth- and early twentieth-century libraries, their rarified style and interior organization worked together to elicit genteel – read: "silent" – behavior from patrons. The New York Public Library was organized with each successive floor containing more public functions, with the top floor devoted entirely to the public. The reading room was placed at the back of the top floor, away from the bustle of Fifth Avenue and near the closed book stacks. The use of open or closed book stacks touches on a long debate over the relationship between patrons and media – what kinds of media should be available, and to whom? – questions that have implications for how the collection should be organized, and what the relationships between patrons, library material and library buildings should *sound* like. Middle-class users, assumed to be the serious "scholars," were protected as much as possible from the "messy realities" and the noise of the staff, less serious working-class patrons and children (Van Slyck 1995: 98–9).

In his study of the Rose Reading Room, Kelman has little opportunity to discuss how the *physical space* itself enforces appropriate behavior – how it functions in the library's disciplinary machine. He wonders how "to best ensure that [the library] – and the people found there – will properly perform?" (Kelman 2001: 30). How, concretely, does this reading room "stage and script" appropriate patron behavior, which here means silent, private reading? Kelman notes the "awesome and imposing structure" and the "large white marble halls [that] amplify even the smallest sound and betray one's 'uncivil' behavior," and describes patrons who are particularly conscious of their noise-making behaviors: pushing in a chair, closing a book, flipping pages (2001: 29, 34–5, 38). We can infer that this sensitivity is a consequence of the room's "live" acoustics, which are themselves a product of the 51-foot ceilings, 78-foot by 297-foot dimensions, the quarry tile on the floors and the weighty wood chairs that stutter when they scrape across them. This room is a literal echo chamber for "uncivil behavior."

At the turn of the twentieth century, library philosophy was changing, as was the design of library buildings and the sounds made in them. "The traditional understanding of the library as a treasure house, protecting its books from untrustworthy readers, was falling out of currency," Van Slyck writes (1995: 25). Open shelves, branch libraries and other forms of outreach, often undertaken in conjunction with other Progressive public services, were making noise. Roughly a third of all libraries included in a 1902 *Architectural Review* survey contained group study rooms, exhibition rooms, lecture halls, club rooms – programmatic areas that were certainly not silent (cited in Van Slyck 1995: 32–3).

Children's libraries provide a striking example of just how "unquiet" the public library may have been. The aforementioned survey showed that by 1902 nearly 75 percent of all libraries had children's rooms. Many of them had entrances separate from the library proper, so as "to ensure that the genteel library user enjoyed the illusion of ordered and serene opulence…" (ibid.: 100). Many Carnegie libraries' children's rooms did employ architectural features – including stylistic references to middle-class homes – to encourage appropriate "inside" behavior. Yet we also find more children's rooms with reading alcoves for storytelling and spaces dedicated to film screenings, puppet programs and other activities that involved the production of sound (ibid.: 186–7). Even if the children's room was sufficiently removed from the library proper to keep the giggles and shouts contained, the room itself was often a noisy place.

Some of that noise was unsanctioned. Children occasionally failed to see the library, as its board undoubtedly did, as a haven from the clamor of the city. Regarding it instead as an "extension of the street," these children brought their outdoor voices indoors. Echoing Lessing and Bailey, Van Slyck suggests that "boisterousness was one of the methods that children used to stake their claim to public space" (ibid.: 213). The noise was a result of the architecture's failure to communicate its message of "decorum" effectively:

> Architecture's transformative powers were limited by the fact that its signals are socially and culturally coded. If many working-class and immigrant children remained untouched by the library's message, it was because the library attempted to

communicate in a language that these young readers did not understand (ibid.: 216).

Some patrons – perhaps those not familiar with the connotations of Beaux Arts and Richardsonian architectural styles, or rationally ordered interiors – failed to perceive the codes of silence supposedly built into the library building.

From Disciplinary Machine to Disciplined Choice

"Previous knowledge of public institutions, attitudes about reading, access to other urban amenities – all of these factors influenced how readers understood their own rights and responsibilities at the public library," Van Slyck writes (1995: 201). Psychologists Henk Aarts and Ap Dijksterhuis confirm her conclusion. They conducted a series of experiments designed to test situational norms – "generally accepted beliefs about how to behave in particular situations (and environments) … [that] are learned by associating normative behavior to these situations" (Aarts and Dijksterhuis 2003: 18). The researchers wondered, "do we keep the level of noise down automatically on the mere activation of the symbolic representation of a library?" (ibid.: 19). They found that "strength of association" was a key independent variable. People with a weak "association" between normative behavior and libraries – those not familiar with the institution or its codes of behavior – were unlikely to know to lower their voices. Thus a patron who has never before set foot in a library – or even a regular patron unaccustomed to libraries built in unfamiliar architectural styles – might find that the building inadequately "stag[es] and script[s]" decorous patron behavior, and may even fail to denote the building type. For instance, will patrons, upon encountering the new glass anvil-shaped Visual and Performing Arts Library in Brooklyn, know how to "read" the building as a library and understand its behavioral script?

Foucauldian models have often been used to describe how libraries "discipline" their patrons, or how professional discourses construct the "administrative power" of librarianship. Library historian Alistair Black notices that it is libraries' "'darker' side that has often attracted critical historical scholarship, the side that is disciplinary, distant, and controlling. The negative dimension … interfaces easily with the work of Michel Foucault" (Black 2005: 418). Yet Foucault has been widely criticized for allowing little room for human agency or resistance – for inadequately accounting for those who fail to read, or intentionally ignore, the institution's "script." Edward Said argues that Foucault confuses "the power of institutions to subjugate individuals" with "the fact that individual behavior in society is frequently a matter of following rules or conventions" – conventions like architecture's culturally coded behavioral cues (1986: 151).[2] Although his later theories of governmentality addressed some of the critiques of his earlier works, Foucault's theories still may not be the best suited to addressing a modern-day institution that has largely abandoned a Progressive agenda of discipline and assimilation. As Harris (1973) argues, the modern-day American public library is no longer an "authoritarian and elitist" institution; the modern institution is a guardian of the "people's right to know" – a role that, he says, requires trusting patrons to know what is best for themselves – and, we can assume, how to behave themselves.[3]

Van Slyck argues that during the Carnegie era, libraries' focus on efficiency and solitary reading led the institution to squander its "potential to serve as a site – literally and figuratively – for public discussion and debate," but the library has since reclaimed that potential (1995: 219). Libraries can be, and often are, sites for debate and resistance – to privatization, social atomization, segregation, commercialization etc. – and it is this potential for resistance, I think, that should compel us to seek more appropriate theoretical models to think about how today's library functions in its civic context, as an institution and for its inhabitants. We need to find new ways to think about the resonance, both figurative and literal, of these buildings. Today, "great public libraries provide a place for not only gathering or storing ideas, but engaging with them," says Nancy Tessman (personal communication, July 20, 2006), Director of the Salt Lake City Public Library, which opened a new central library in 2003. "That process may create some noise. Our objective is to enable and encourage the engagement while still providing places of relative quiet for reading and musing. Good design will allow a reasonable mixture of both." It seems that today's libraries are not as hostile toward noise as their recent ancestors were – not because noise has ceased to be a problem, but because librarians and architects realize that silence, although beneficial or necessary for some of the activities that take place in the library, is not the ideal condition for *all* programmatic elements. "We didn't set out to be an 'Unquiet Library,'" Tessman says. "We just recognized that learning and communicating have changed over the decades, and 'quiet' is not the main objective."

Schafer advocates for the "recovery of positive silence." Most contemporary public libraries offer this: silence as a *choice*. The more we acknowledge the ability of patrons to choose how to use the library, the better prepared we are to think about the library as providing a field of possibilities, behavioral and acoustic, for its users. And the more likely we are to realize that Foucault's models may not be the best suited for thinking critically and constructively about today's library. Bourdieu's notion of *habitus* was central to Sterne's work, and I believe it will serve us well here. Bourdieu defines habitus ([1972] 1990: 72) as the system of "durable, transposable dispositions, structured structures predisposed to function as structuring structures," that is, as principles which generate and organize practices and representations that can be objectively adapted to their outcomes without presupposing a conscious aiming at ends of an express mastery of the operations necessary in order to attain them. Objectively "regulated" and "regular" without being in any way the product of obedience to rules, they can be collectively orchestrated without being the product of the organizing action of a conductor ([1972] 1990: 72).

The concept of habitus allows us to address the *orchestration* of sound in space, not its control. It does not presuppose mastery of, or even conscious familiarity with, normative behaviors or the spatial codes assumed to elicit them. Further, habitus deals with predispositions rather than reflexes; it allows us to address the fact that our responses to architecture and media are not automatic, instinctual. It acknowledges a structure, but allows for choice and variation, without supposing that that choice is limitless; the library is not anarchic. If a patron behaves, or "sounds out," in a way that is outside the "structuring structures" of a particular space in the library, he may be directed to an area that is more appropriate for his behavior.

Finally, as Sterne notes, the concept of the habitus enables us to explore a "mix of custom, bodily technique, social outlook, style, and orientation" – a mix similar to the variables that, as we have seen, shape people's perceptions of and reactions to noise and architecture (2003: 92). The customs, techniques, postures and styles through which people interact with one another and with media are shaped by the social spaces, or *fields*, in which those interactions take place – and are the proper concern of architectural design. As Jean Hillier and Emma Rooksby write in their introduction to *Habitus: A Sense of Place*,

> Comprehension of agents' habituses, influencing their tendencies to act in particular manners, their motivations, preferences, worldviews, aspirations and expectations, will ... enable better improvisation and navigation around the complexities of the social practices which constitute planning processes (2005: 12–13).

The dispositions and practices that constitute the habitus do not, unlike Sterne's "audile techniques," imply conscious, rational choice. "The habitus is not cognitively understood but rather internalized and embodied," architect Kim Dovey writes (2005: 283–97 at 284). Designing in light of the *habitus* of listening and looking, of what we will call the conditions of attendance – visual, haptic and sonic – to particular media, does not mean prescribing certain patron behaviors. It does not mean promoting the "one best" practice of listening or the "one best sound." Rather, it means creating a field of what Bourdieu calls "possibles," or potentials of interaction between people, media and architecture. Examining the library as an acoustic space requires that we adjoin Sterne and Thompson – that we think about the various technologies of listening and the audile techniques they promote, as we also consider how those technologies function within, and interact with, the architecture that houses them.

Sonic Spatial Organization through Site and Program

At the most macroscopic level of analysis, we see that even the placement of libraries within their urban contexts has acoustic implications. Today's downtown libraries, unlike those sited in accordance with City Beautiful principles, are often positioned to serve as anchors of vibrant areas of mixed-use development, and they usually have their own stops on metropolitan bus lines or light rail systems. This new civic position brings the noise of commerce and transportation right to the library's doors. Many of these "destination" libraries, designed by high-profile architects, draw thousands of patrons whose primary purpose is to gawk and snap photos; their presence – their footsteps, voices and camera clicks – must be planned for, as well.

It seems that acoustics has only recently become a separate, explicit concern in library design. In the past, "sound" issues were often folded into broader interests, like traffic control and surveillance. In a 1941 library planning book the index entry for "Acoustics" reads, "see Noise Reduction," suggesting that the primary concern was keeping unwanted sound *out* – not designing for those sounds that were desirable or germane to the activity taking place inside the building (Wheeler and Githens 1941). This is what Schafer refers to as a shift from "positive to negative acoustic design" – a shift toward designing *against*, rather than designing *for* – in early- to mid-twentieth-century modern architecture. Today's architects practice a mix of both kinds of acoustic design: some use masking, or soundproofing, to cover up noises – while others use materials that can freely resonate, or create spaces that facilitate or flatter the sounds produced by the space's activity.[4]

Today's designers often integrate sounds that were once designed *out* (although not necessarily *kept* out) of the library. Sounds of human activity, and speech in particular, are regarded as germane to the central functions of the library and are thus planned for.[5] The library has also taken on new functions, some commercial, that produce sounds that must be "orchestrated" into the library soundscape. Many consultants have recommended separating lobbies – which are where these multipurpose functions are sometimes housed – from the library proper. The Salt Lake City Public Library, designed by Moshe Safdie, heeded this advice. In Figure 2 we see the library's Urban Room, a vibrant multifunctional space that is separate from the library proper and that serves as its oversized foyer. A vertical "reading room," offering alcoves with spaces for both individual and

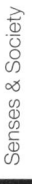

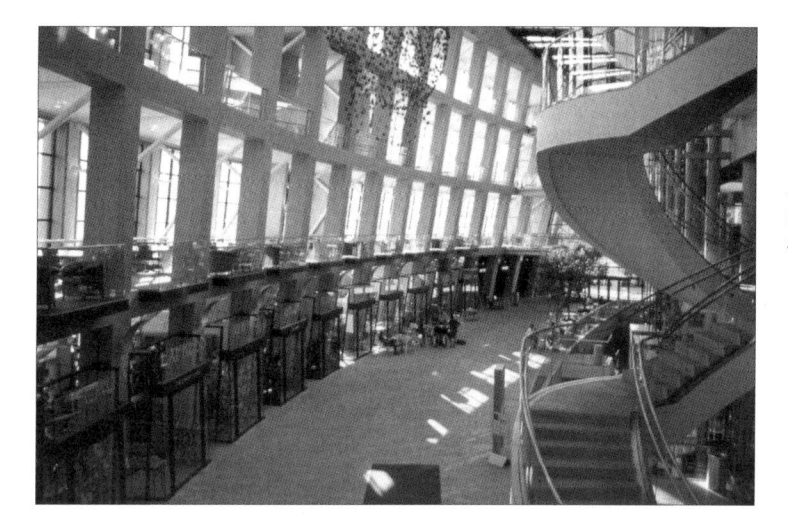

Figure 2
Salt Lake City's Urban Room. Photograph by S. Mattern.

group work, is accessible via bridges that traverse the Urban Room. The room succeeds as a vibrant public space – but, in orchestrating a habitus for study, this arrangement seems disconcerting: in order to gain entry to a space for quiet, silent reading, one must cross a cavern of commerce with footsteps echoing from the stone floor below.

One technique that many designers employ during programming, and that helps to ensure the most effective organization of the library's acoustic environments, is an "acoustical grouping" or hierarchizing of sonic spaces. Salt Lake City's program (see Figure 3) recommended that the building's spaces fall on a gradient of privacy and publicity, including fully enclosed, secure spaces, semitransparent spaces and fully open spaces (RPG Partnership 1999: i). The New York Public Library, you will recall, adopted a similar strategy: each successive floor contained more public areas, with the top floor devoted almost entirely to public functions. Today, many library planners combine functionally- and acoustically-"like" functions (see Figure 4), hierarchizing private and public, hushed and vibrant, closed and open spaces. They often specify that the high-activity, high-noise public activities be placed off major circulation corridors or close to the building's main entrance on the ground floor, while "serious" research areas are placed farther away.

Yet, some designers have failed to effectively program patrons' listening experiences. When it first opened in 2001, the renovated New York Public Library for the Performing Arts at Lincoln Center featured a central reading room that opened onto a bank of elevators and a photocopy room, and was adjacent to service desks where patrons retrieved materials. As the *New York Times*' Joseph Horowitz wrote,

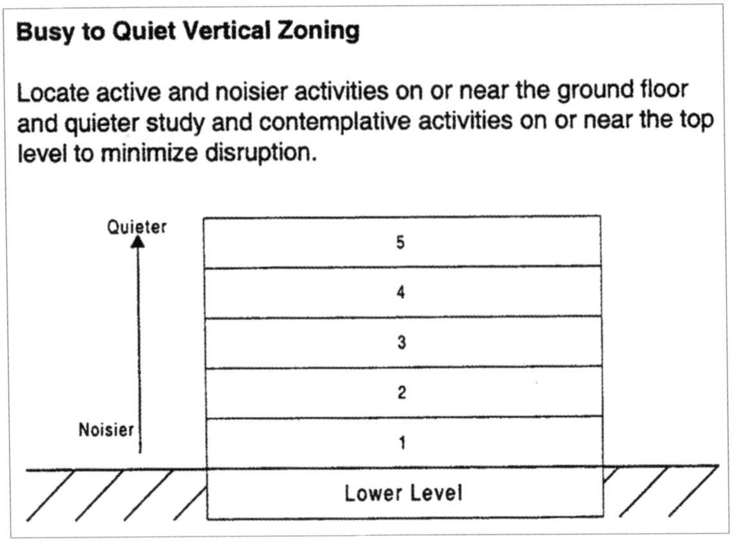

Figure 3
Salt Lake City's building program called for a gradient of sound throughout the building's floors, with louder, more public functions near the ground level and quieter, private functions in the upper levels. Photograph courtesy of Resource Planning Group (RPG) Inc.

Busy to Quiet Vertical Zoning

Locate active and noisier activities on or near the ground floor and quieter study and contemplative activities on or near the top level to minimize disruption.

The array of undesired noise plays a practical joke on traditional sensitivities. The metallic clang of the doors to the stacks, the resonant footfall of elevator passengers, ... the reprimands at the security station ... – more than audible, all these sounds are italicized in the exposed low-ceilinged space with its 46 video playback stations, 12 audio stations and 30 computerized workstations. (2002: B31)

Far from offering spaces of sonic "closure," this library was beset with acoustic leaks. And where the building itself failed to provide cues about its appropriate use, human monitors had to step in with verbal directives, which only further contributed to the clamor and confusion. The library has since undergone further renovation to correct these acoustical problems.

Designing the Listening Experience

Designing the sonic experience of a library is not just a matter of deciding what goes where. It involves a particular sensitivity to the *kind* and *quality* of media interactions and learning experiences that take place in a library. Because Kelman's case is unique – the Rose Reading Room is devoted primarily to *books* and their *silent*, private consumption – he has no opportunity to address encounters with a diversity of media or diverse practices of reading. Yet observation in many modern-day library buildings reveals myriad practices of reading: solitary, partnered or collective; silent, aloud or accompanied by a musical soundtrack; upright, seated or prone; indoors or outdoors. So, while private, contemplative reading does benefit from silence, this is only one of many reading practices – some of which either produce sound or thrive in its presence. Plus, patrons can read – and *listen to* and *screen* and *navigate* – media in many formats. So when Kelman writes that "[at] the library it does not matter quite what one reads, but how," that "what" necessarily refers in his case to books. Elsewhere we cannot make such assumptions – and it is the *what* that determines the *how*. Specific media forms require specific practices of consumption – specific visual or "audile" techniques.

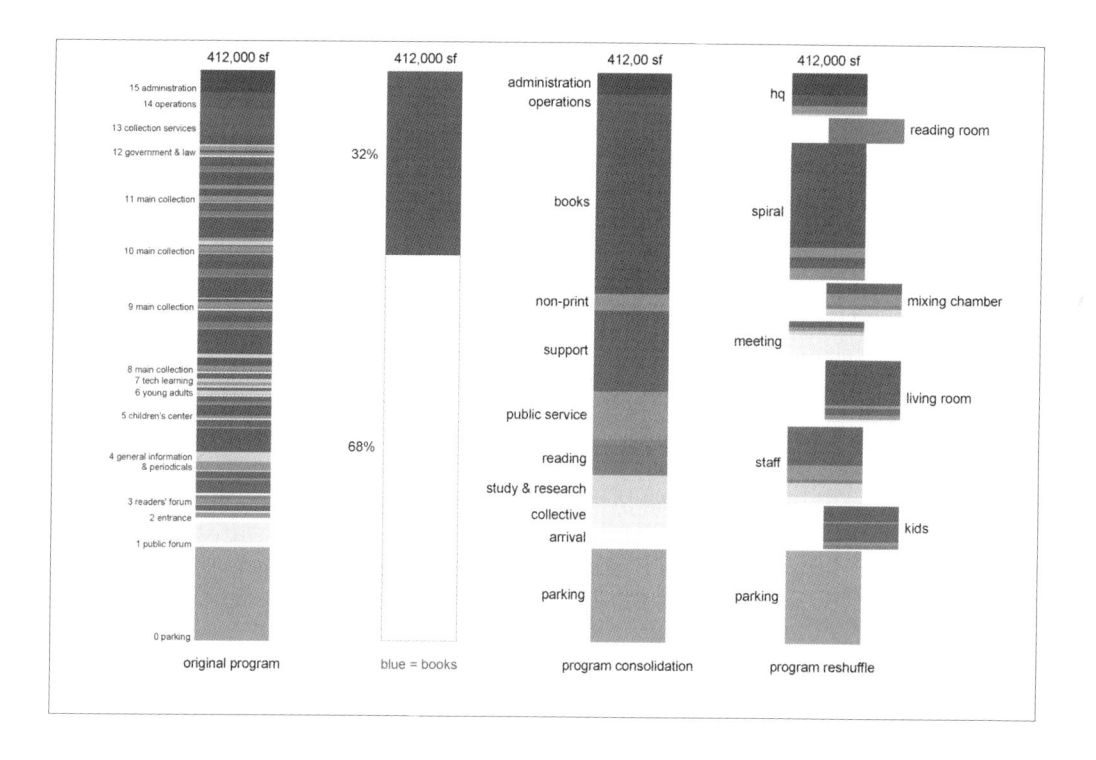

Sterne's concept of "audile technique" can shed light on these interactions and experiences – but his terminology may not be ideal for informing design decisions. The term "technique" implies intention and rationality, as Sterne acknowledges. But not all listening is intentional and rational; it is occasionally accidental, irrational, nonlinear – and these varied practices of listening all have a place in the library. A concept perhaps more readily and effectively translated into responsive design – designing in light of the habitus of media reception – is what Joshua Meyrowitz refers to as "conditions of attendance" (1985: 84–91).[6] "Conditions of attendance" refer to the conditions – environmental, situational, emotional, sensory etc. – under which one "attends to" a particular medium. The assumption is that different media forms necessitate or benefit from particular conditions in which they can be accessed and attended to. Reading a book, for instance, calls for adequate lighting, while viewing a

Figure 4
In Seattle, the architects itemized all the types of activities, or programmatic functions, that take place in a library, then combined the "like" functions – and allowed this grouping to inform the shape of the building. Photograph courtesy of the Office for Metropolitan Architecture (OMA).

projected film calls for darkness. Solitary reading requires relative silence, although some collaborative reading – like a mother reading to her child, or an ESL teacher and student working together – introduces sound into the environment. Even the physical posture and the degree of mental engagement one must assume vary by medium, and these qualities, too, are influenced by the space in which a medium is accessed.

But according to Geoffrey Freeman (personal communication, May 15, 2003) of Shepley Bulfinch Richardson and Abbott, a firm with an impressive library design resumé, many of today's library users engage with texts without noting the format in which they appear. As the Office for Metropolitan Architecture (OMA), designers of the Seattle library, acknowledged, library planners need to create spaces that facilitate the use of multiple media, perhaps simultaneously (see Figure 5). "In an age where (*sic*) information can be accessed anywhere," the architects write, "it is the simultaneity of all media and the professionalism of their presentation and interaction, that will make the Library new" (1999: 7). The library, if it is to remain relevant, has to fashion itself into a "one stop" media center. But the library is not a warehouse; these media, as OMA acknowledges, must be thoughtfully, "professionally" presented in a way that takes into account their format-specific needs and facilitates patrons' interactions with them and their interaction with one another.

Still, many libraries continue to use – and in fact many have recently instituted – format-*defined* departments. Many have an audiovisual (A/V) department (see Figure 6), and most have placed

Figure 5 Media Types
The Office for Metropolitan Architecture, designers of the Seattle Public Library, map the proliferation of media types that the library is obligated to accommodate. Photograph courtesy of the Office for Metropolitan Architecture (OMA)

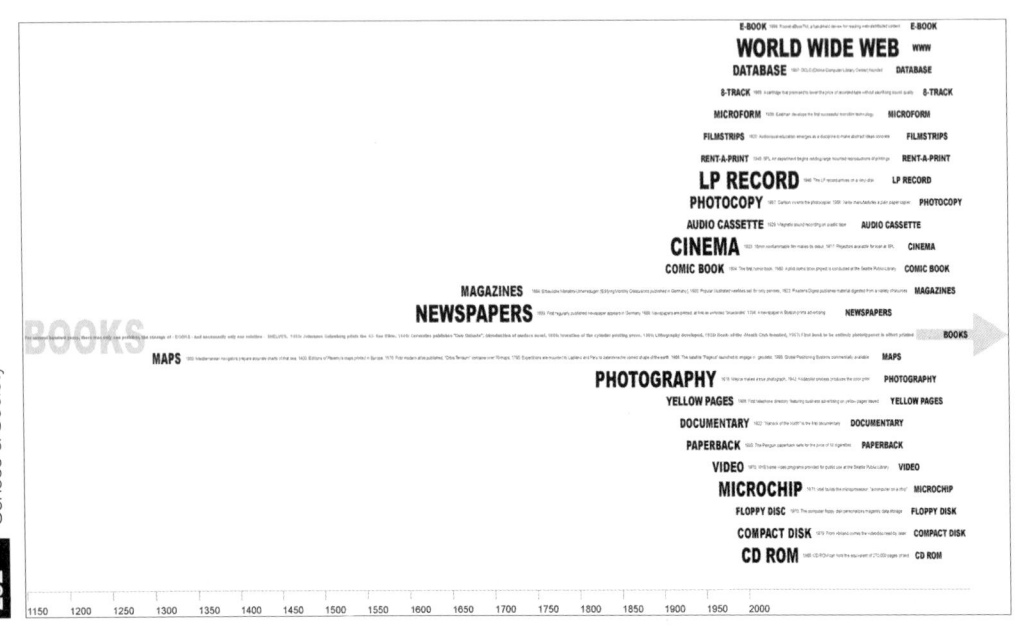

those collections near their buildings' front entrances because, as the Toledo library's administration has realized, A/V people are not always book people, and they should not have to traverse a building full of books to pick up a video or CD. Several libraries have adopted similar strategies. But, by exiling the compact discs and DVDs to the first floor – often many floors away from the books whose content they share – libraries are physically as well as intellectually, pedagogically and ideologically separating these media, defining A/V materials as *popular* materials and books as *research* materials.

Varying conditions of attendance have also foiled these attempts to integrate media formats. Libraries continue to face the challenge of finding appropriate listening and viewing spaces (see Figure 7). As Salt Lake City planned its new building, librarians hoped that new listening and viewing technologies – something more efficient and secure than the existing technology – would come along. But when that failed to happen, the library settled for individual preview rooms where patrons can listen to audio or watch video recordings. Most buildings, likewise, promote solitary listening and viewing – but Phoenix's Burton Barr Central Library, in its teen room, has inserted a group exhibition area, where films are shown after school to teenagers lounging in bean bags. The space – designed by the teenagers themselves, in cooperation with architect Will Bruder – reflects an impressive sensitivity to the teenage habitus of viewing – one that is more informal, communal and perhaps a bit more distracted. Teen Central occupies a corner of the library's fourth floor,

Figure 6
San Antonio, like many libraries, has separated its audiovisual collection from the print collection, and placed it in a separately secured area easily accessible from the front entrance to the library. Photograph by S. Mattern.

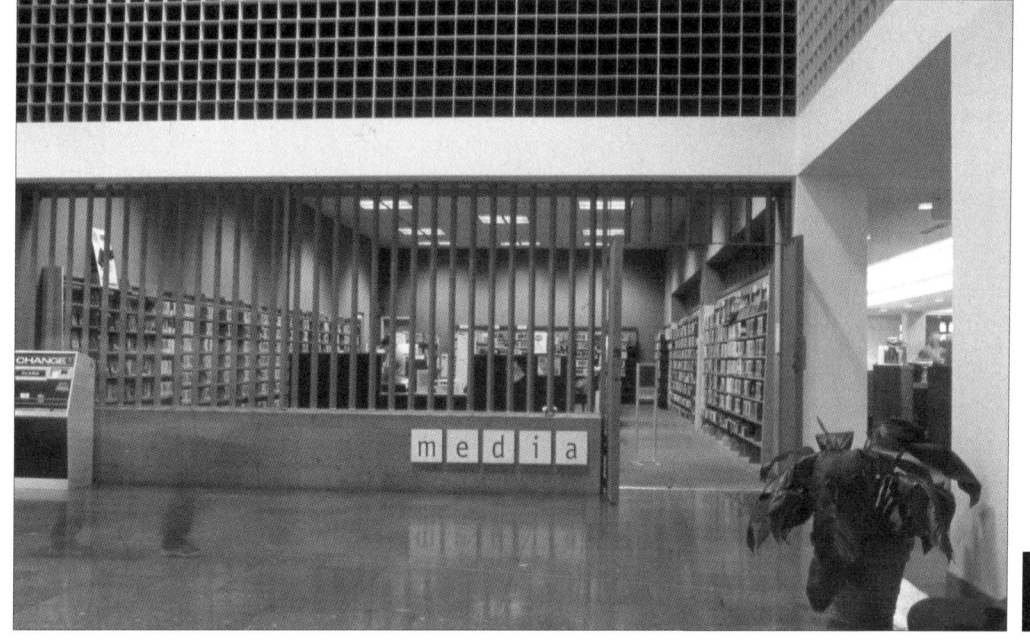

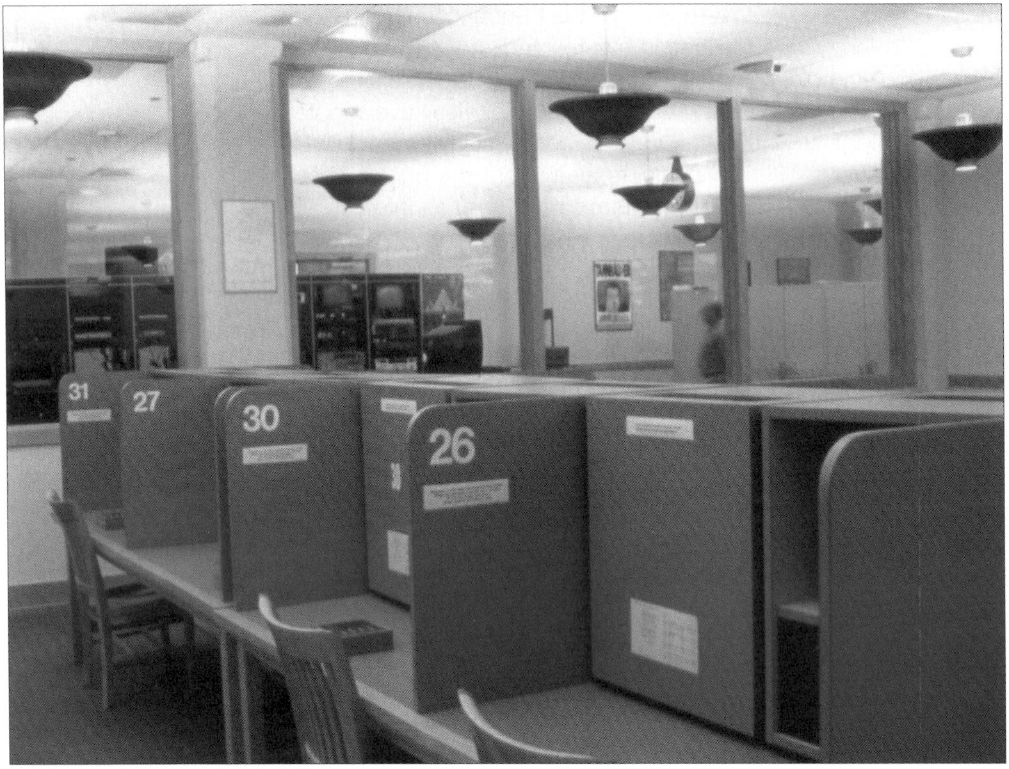

Figure 7
In Chicago, as in other libraries, listening and viewing activities are given dedicated spaces, which usually offer little in the way of aesthetics or comfort. Photograph by S. Mattern.

which it shares with rather unlikely partners: the rare book room and the Arizona Room for special collections. Only on rare occasions, "when we have the music up really loud," does sound permeate the sound-resistant wall between it and the Arizona Room next door – transforming the *music* into *noise* – a teen librarian said.

The necessity for different access technologies and different conditions for media reception – such as viewing and listening stations, which are difficult, if not impossible, to integrate throughout the building – means that certain kinds of media are necessarily concentrated in media-specific departments. Until new technology allows for the integration of listening (and viewing) stations throughout the stacks – until HyperSonic™ Sound, or focused speakers, keep the movie soundtrack from leaking into the stacks and distracting nearby readers, or until A/V planners can find a way to provide secure, sanitary earphones for patrons to listen to the audio books shelved among the traditional tomes – library planners may have to shelve their plans for a "format-blind" organization.[7] In the meantime, planners might focus on thinking *experientially* about patrons' interactions with media and appropriate sonic "conditions of attendance." Brian Lang of the British Library writes about these conditions in terms of "relationships":

An obvious one is the relationship between the library building and the readers. Other key relationships are those between readers and the library's collections, between readers and librarians, between librarians and the collection, and between the collection and the building (1999: 11–24 at 12).

What might these relationships *sound* like? How do both people and media make the architecture *resonate*? How is the ear engaged when a book falls from a high shelf onto a metal floor, or when the hum emanating from a pod of copy machines invades an otherwise peaceful reading room? What are the poetics of these breaches of spatial closure?

In Seattle, the architects and librarians realized that patrons have a dynamic relationship with print materials – and that there is no single sound of reading. The designers placed atop the building a huge, vaulting, reading room (see Figure 8). It is important to note that even in designs that pride themselves on their technological progressiveness, such as Seattle's, reading is usually hosted in the building's most majestic spaces. And perhaps rightly so. These spaces, with their chandeliers and ample sunlight, are well suited for a medium whose surface is reflective rather than transmitted, and whose presentation of content, more so than that of time-based media, allows for *reflection*, an act deserving a dignified space.

Within the room are different conditions, from the intimate and informal to the rigorous and organized, from linearly ordered carrels to grouped side chairs, for all kinds of reading moods, methods and materials. Even if different arrangements and postures of reading are permitted, this is still to be a *quiet* space. Architecturally, the space

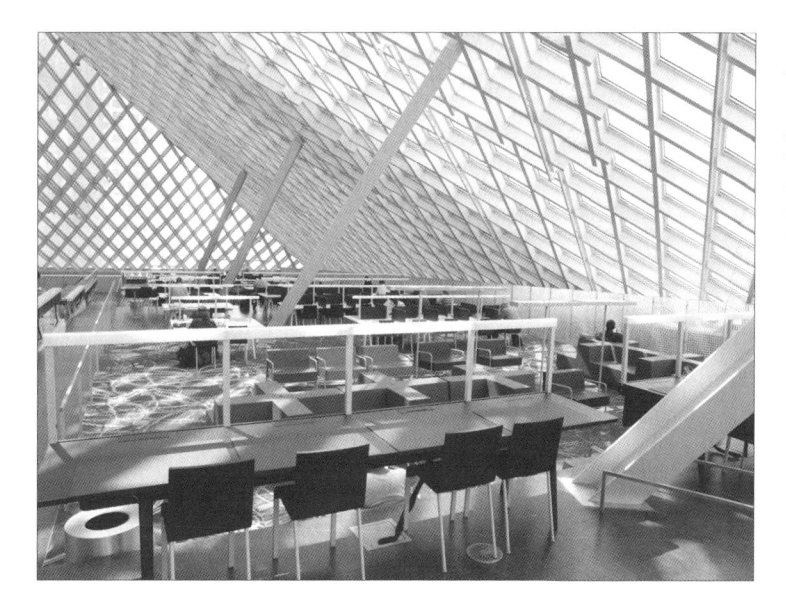

Figure 8
The Seattle Public Library's Reading Gallery offers an amphitheatrical space, with myriad seating arrangements, for quiet media use. Photograph by Mark Anunson.

is "driven by glass," acoustical designer Basel Jurdy noted, and the only sound-absorptive materials are the white "pillows" (see Figure 9) along the sides and on the underside of the tenth-floor ceiling. But, even with the pillows in place, the reading room is still "lively" – not an ideal condition for a quiet reading space. Yet, Jurdy (personal communication, January 13, 2006) explains, the reading room "can still be okay acoustically if people aren't carrying on conversations to excite the acoustical anomalies" of the space. In other words, if patrons somehow pick up design cues or "situational norms" indicating that this is a *quiet* reading space and behave accordingly – if the space itself sets the appropriate habitus, if they observe that other patrons are working quietly – then the room's potential brightness need not be an issue. But, as I have witnessed in a few buildings, if a patron is clicking away on his laptop in an area that the patrons themselves have defined, through practice, as a quiet study zone, he is likely to be asked politely by one of those silent studiers to move to an area where his clicking will not be perceived as "noise."

That more sonically tolerant space is Seattle's ground-floor "living room" – an informal alternative to the reading room (see Figure 10). The space's proximity to the fiction collection, the cafe and the library store, and its provision of a variety of work areas and

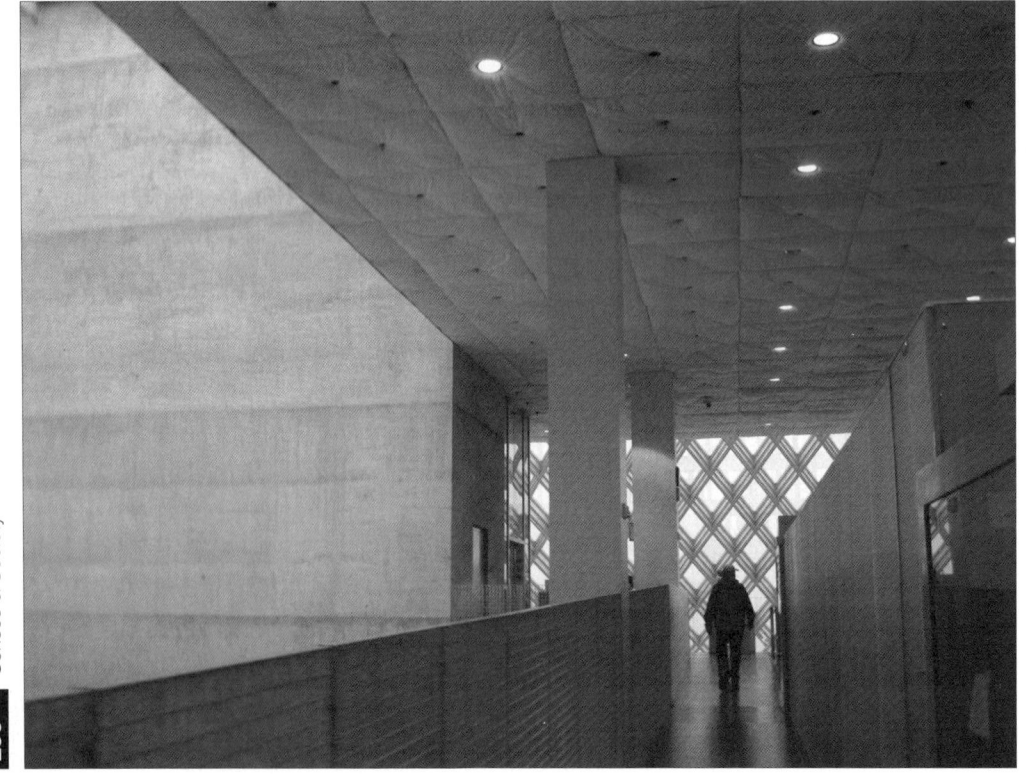

Figure 9
White "pillows" help to absorb sound in the quiet reading room of the Seattle Public Library, where the building materials would otherwise make for a highly reverberant space. Photograph courtesy of Emily Lin

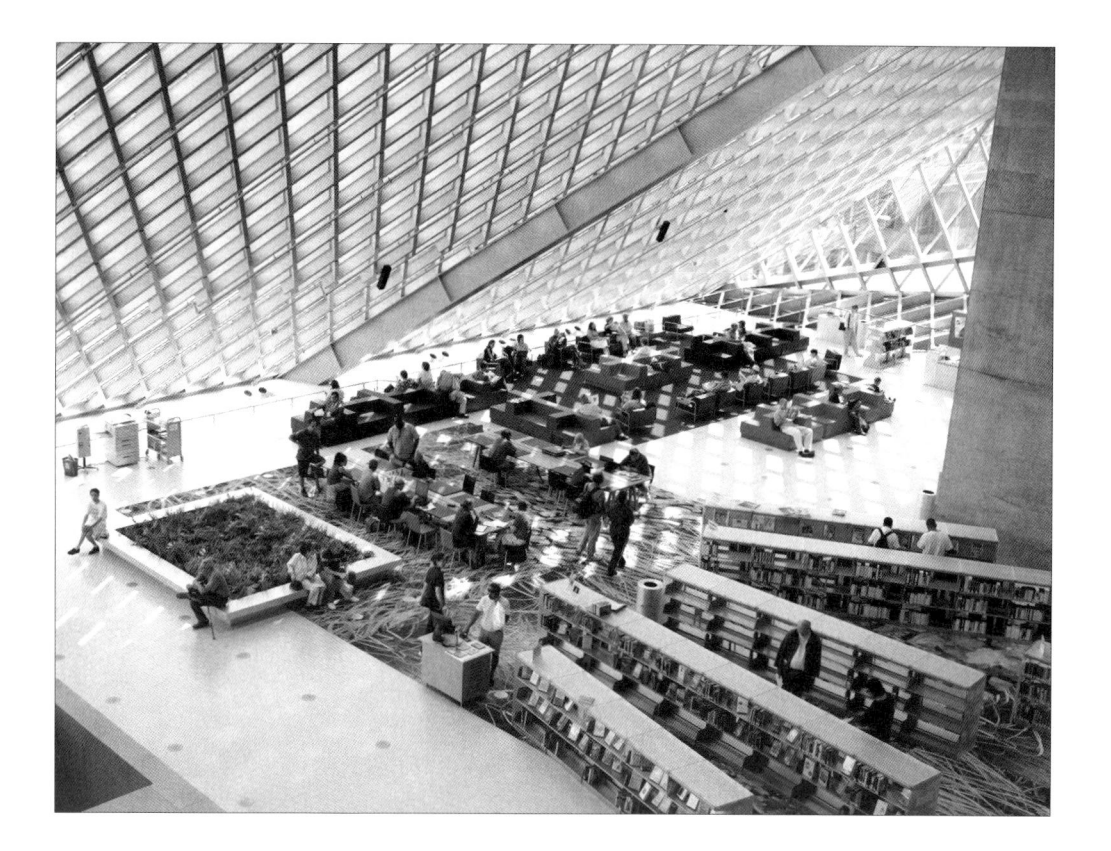

Figure 10
Seattle's "living room" provides space for louder, more social kinds of work with media. This space also features a café and the library shop. Photograph by Mark Anunson.

seating arrangements, orients patrons toward a more collaborative, "sounded" style of reading and working. Its purpose, Jurdy says, "is to attract people to sit and read or converse"; in order to do this, the space has to be "warm acoustically, but not too reverberant." The area's walls are all glass, a highly reverberant material – but here the glass is canted, which allows the area's "acoustical energy" to bounce to the other floors that open onto the living room, and thus dampen the sound a bit – just enough to allow for reading, while not being so oppressively silent as to deter conversation. Thus, once again, as in the living room, this space creates particular conditions of attendance, which, in turn, affect visitors' perceptions of, and interactions with, media and architecture. Finishes, furnishings and a host of other design cues work together to structure the range of possible behaviors, to establish a habitus appropriate for the function of the space.[8]

Freeman, discussing his experience in designing academic libraries, notes that "it is important to accommodate the sound of learning – lively group discussions or intense conversations over coffee – while controlling the impact of acoustics on surrounding space." At the same time, "we must never lose sight of the dedicated, contemplative spaces that will remain an important aspect of any place of scholarship" (2005: n.p.) There is room – there is *need* – for both acoustic conditions ... and plenty in between.

Accommodating this variety is not a matter of *controlling* acoustics or *disciplining* listeners. In designing a library, one cannot expect to use architecture to regulate people and the sounds that they and their media make. Rather, accommodating acoustics are developed from the ground up, by looking at how people, media and architecture relate, and then using architectural design to facilitate their meaningful interaction. Considering the sounds of human presence, the sounds of media, the sounds of building materials, and how these various sounds interact; considering how various acoustic zones should be positioned in relation to one another; considering the visual, haptic and *sonic* environments – the conditions of attendance – most appropriate for various activities; considering what practices and postures of listening and learning the library intends to promote – all of these are issues that, if considered early during the programming and schematic design phases and not forgotten during design development, can inform the design of libraries that *sound* like the dynamic, responsive, culturally resonant institutions that today's libraries strive to be.

Acknowledgments

I owe much gratitude to the organizers and attendees of the Architecture | Music | Acoustics conference in Toronto in June 2006; and to Barry Salmon, Kevin Allen, and the students in our Sound & Space class, taught at The New School in the fall of 2005. Thanks, too, to Marita Surken, Lance Strate, Curtis Marez, Michael Bull, and the anonymous reviewers of this article.

Notes

1. See Bijsterveld, 2001, 2003; Schafer, 1977: 181–202; Smilor, 1977; Thompson, 2002: 115-68.
2. See Eco, Umberto. 1986. "Functionalism and Sign: The Semiotics of Architecture." In Mark Gottdiener and A. Lagopoulos [ed.] *The City and the Sign*. New York: Columbia University Press: 56-85.
3. Critics might argue that in light of the contemporary "War on Terror" and the Patriot Act, *laissez-faire* librarianship is now only a memory of a more innocent past. I do not mean to trivialize the serious and deleterious consequences, both for individuals and for libraries, of these political developments. Still, I disagree with those who regard the contemporary library as a (remodeled) disciplinary machine – a government-controlled surveillance mechanism, although one now more Deleuzian than Foucauldian. The federal government may intend to use library borrowing records and Internet search histories to identify would-be terrorists, but the American Library Association (2003) publicly "opposes any use of governmental power to suppress the free and open exchange of knowledge and information or to intimidate individuals exercising

free inquiry" (n.p.). What is more, the library building itself it still designed primarily through a partnership between librarians and architects, both of whom are generally committed to upholding the institution's core contemporary values of access and empowerment.
4. See Salter, C.M. n.d.; Scherer J. 2001; Wrightson D. and Wrightson, J.M. 1999.
5. Given and Leckie (2003), in a study mapping the social activity of two Canadian public libraries, noted that, although talking has traditionally been discouraged in the library, "talking as a behavior was often part of the patrons' generally studious activities." "Given the popularity of talking among the users observed in this study, the need for areas conducive to talk need (sic) to be factored into library-design" (382).
6. Meyrowitz, who studied in the doctoral program in Media Ecology at New York University, was undoubtedly inspired by the unpublished works of Christine Nystrom.
7. The teen library at the new Minneapolis Public Library, opened in the spring of 2006, includes directed speakers that allow groups to listen to music without bothering nearby patrons. Its effectiveness has yet to be seen.
8. Architectural critic Lawrence Cheek (2007) complains that the Living Room "harvests and energizes routine noise," rendering it "not conducive to intimacy with a book" (Lawrence Cheek, (2007). "On Architecture: How the New Central Library Really Stacks Up" *Seattle Post-Intelligencer* (March 27): http://seattlepi.nwsource.com/ae/309029_architecture27.html?source=mypi).

References

Aarts, Henck and Dijksterhuis, Ap. 2003. "The Silence of the Library: Environment, Situational Norm, and Social Behavior," *Journal of Personality and Social Psychology*, 84 (1): 18–28.

American Library Association. 2003. Resolution on the USA Patriot Act and Related Measures That Infringe on the Rights of Library Users. 2003 ALA Midwinter Meeting, Philadelphia, PA (January 29): http://www.ala.org/ala/washoff/WOissues/civilliberties/theusapatriotact/alaresolution.htm (accessed August 1, 2006).

Bailey, Peter. 1996. "Breaking the Sound Barrier: A Historian Listens to Noise," *Body & Society*, 3 (2): 49–66.

Baron, Lawrence. 1982. "Noise and Degeneration: Theodor Lessing's Crusade for Quiet," *Journal of Contemporary History*, 17 (1): 165–78.

Bijsterveld, Karin. 2001. "The Diabolical Symphony of the Mechanical Age: Technology and Symbolism of Sound in European and North American Noise Abatement Campaigns, 1900–40," *Social Studies of Science*, 34 (1): 37–70.

——. 2003. "'The City of Din': Decibels, Noise, and Neighbors in the Netherlands, 1910–1980," *Osiris*, 18: 173–93.

Black, Alistair. 2005. "The Library as Clinic: A Foucauldian Interpretation of British Public Library Attitudes to Social and Physical Disease, ca. 1850–1950," *Libraries & Culture*, 40 (3): 416–34.

Bourdieu, Pierre. 1977. *Outline of a Theory of Practice*. Cambridge: Cambridge University Press.

——. 1990. *The Logic of Practice*. Cambridge: Polity Press.

Clark, J. W. 1894. *Libraries in the Medieval and Renaissance Periods*. Chicago: Argonaut.

Demas, Sam. 2005. "From the Ashes of Alexandria: What's Happening in the College Library?" In Council on Library and Information Resources [ed.] *Library as Place: Rethinking Roles, Rethinking Space*. Washington, DC: Council on Library and Information Resources (February): http://www.clir.org/pubs/reports/pub129/demas.html (accessed July 5, 2006).

Dovey, Kim. (2005). "The Silent Complicity of Architecture," In Jean Hillier and Emma Rooksby (eds), *Habitus: A Sense of Place* (2nd edn). Burlington, VT: Ashgate: 283–96.

Freeman, Geoffrey T. 2005. "The Library as Place: Changes in Learning Patterns, Collections, Technology, and Use." In Council on Library and Information Resources [ed.] *Library as Place: Rethinking Roles, Rethinking Space*. Washington, DC: Council on Library and Information Resources (February): http://www.clir.org/PUBS/reports/pub129/freeman.html (accessed July 6, 2006).

Given, Lisa M. and Leckie, Gloria J. 2003. "'Sweeping' the Library: Mapping the Social Activity Space of the Public Library," *Library and Information Science Research*, 25 (4): 385–85.

Harris, Michael. 1973. "The Purpose of the American Public Library: A Revisionist Interpretation of History," *Library Journal* (September 15): 2509–14.

Hillier Jean and Rooksby, Emma (eds). 2005. *Habitus: A Sense of Place* (2nd edn). Burlington, VT: Ashgate.

Hilmes, Michelle. 2005. "Is There a Field Called Sound Culture Studies? And Does It Matter? Review of *The Audible Past: Cultural Origins of Sound Reproduction*, by Jonathan Sterne, and *The Soundscape of Modernity: Architectural Acoustics and the Culture of Listening in America, 1900 to 1930*, by Emily Thompson," *American Quarterly*, 57: 249–59.

Horowitz, Joseph. 2002. "Quiet, Please: This is a Library After All," *New York Times* (January 27): B31.

Kelman, Ari. 2001. "The Sound of the Civic: Reading Noise at the New York Public Library," *American Studies*, 42 (3): 23–41.

Lang, Brian. 1999. "Library Buildings for the New Millennium," In Marie-France Bisbrouck and Marc Chauveinc (eds) *Intelligent Library Buildings: Proceedings of the Tenth Seminar of the International Federation of Library Associations and Institutions,*

The Hague, Netherlands, August 24–29 1997, Section on Library Buildings and Equipment. Munich, Germany: K. G. Saur.

Manguel, Alberto. 1996. *A History of Reading*. New York: Penguin.

Mattern, Shannon. 2007. *The New Downtown Library: Designing With Communities*. Minneapolis: University of Minnesota Press.

Meyrowitz, Joshua. 1985. *No Sense of Place: The Impact of Electronic Media on Social Behavior*. New York: Oxford University Press.

Oehlerts, Donald. E. 1991. *Books and Blueprints: Building America's Public Libraries*. New York: Greenwood Press.

Office for Metropolitan Architecture/LMN. 1999. *Seattle Public Library Proposal*, concept book. Seattle: Authors.

Ong, Walter J. 1982. *Orality and Literacy: The Technologizing of the Word*. New York: Methuen.

RPG Partnership, The. 1999. *Seattle Public Library Facility Program*. Seattle, WA: Author.

Said, Edward. W. 1986. "Foucault and the Imagination of Power," In David Couzens Hoy (ed.) *Foucault: A Critical Reader*. Oxford: Basil Blackwell: 149–55.

Salter, C.M. (n.d.). "Acoustics for Libraries," *Libris design project*, www.librisdesign.org, 3.

Schafer, Murray. 1977. *The Soundscape: Our Sonic Environment and the Tuning of the World*. Rochester, VT: Destiny Books.

Scherer J. 2001. "The Acoustical Environment: Changes and Strategies." Paper presented at the American Library Association Annual Conference, Improving Library Acoustics Workshop, Washington, DC, June 26–30. http://www.msrltd.com/lectures_writings/speeches/ppframe.htm.

Schwartz, Hillel. 2004. "On Noise." In Mark Smith (ed.) *Hearing History: A Reader*. Athens: University of Georgia Press: 51–3.

Seattle Public Library. 2000. *Rem Koolhaas: Seattle library Architecture Design Presentation* [Video] (May 3): Available from the Seattle Public Library, Seattle, WA.

Smilor, Raymond. W. 1977. "Cacophony at 34th Street and 6th: The Noise Problem in America, 1900–1930," *American Studies*, 18 (1): 23–38.

Sterne, Jonathan. 2003. *The Audible Past: Cultural Origins of Sound Reproduction*. Durham, NC: Duke University Press.

Thompson, Emily. 2002. *The Soundscape of Modernity: Architectural Acoustics and the Culture of Listening in America, 1900 to 1930*. Cambridge, MA: MIT Press.

Tisdale, Sally. 1997. "Silence, Please: The Public Library as Entertainment Center," *Harper's Magazine* (March): 65–74.

Van Slyck, Abigail. 1995. *Free to All: Carnegie Libraries & American Culture, 1890–1920*. Chicago: University of Chicago Press.

Wheeler Joseph L. and Githens, Alfred M. 1941. *The American Public Library Building: Its Planning and Design with Special*

Reference to its Administration and Service. Chicago: American Library Association.
Whitehill, Walter Muir. 1956. *Boston Public Library: A Centennial History*. Cambridge: Harvard University Press.
Wrightson D. and Wrightson, J. M. 1999. "Acoustical Considerations in Planning and Design of Library Facilities. *Library Hi Tech*, 17,(4): 349–57.

In Search of Sound: Authenticity, Healing and Redemption in the Early Modern State

Penelope Gouk

Penelope Gouk is a senior lecturer in history at the University of Manchester currently writing about medical explanations of music's effects c. 1500–1750. She is editor of *Musical Healing in Cultural Contexts* and (with Helen Hills) *Representing Emotions*.
gouk@manchester.ac.uk

ABSTRACT   This article is a contribution to early modern sound studies, from the perspective of intellectual history. In contrast to the way visual culture has been handled, few scholars in this field have considered sound in general, or even music in particular, as an agent of change, despite the wealth of scholarship available. Starting with Francis Bacon's ambitious plan to construct a total history of sound--an enterprise ultimately designed to improve the human condition--this paper surveys a series of early modern experiments to recover an authentic golden past, to restore harmony to a chaotic present world, and to heal and restore the soul. It draws on recent as well as more canonical studies in the history of science, early music history and ethnomusicology to suggest how attending to sound can enrich our understanding of the early modern state.

KEYWORDS: music; sound history; experiment; healing; early modern

> Music is the practical knowledge of playing and singing, consisting of sound and song... Their sound, since it is a thing of the senses, both flows away into past time and is impressed on the memory... Unless these sounds are held in the memory by man, they perish, for they cannot be written down.
>
> (Isidore, *Etymologies*)

Western scholarship has come a long way since Isidore dismissed the possibility of recording music back in the seventh century.[1] Over the thousand years between his encyclopedic attempt to organize learning and Francis Bacon's new system of knowledge production, developed in the early 1600s, scholastically-trained composers had invented and refined a notational system capable of representing proportional relationships in both pitch space and time.[2] The earliest forms of musical notation were only an *aide-mémoire*, enabling the reproduction of sounds that were already "impressed on the memory," but after the invention of staff notation in the early eleventh century it eventually became possible not only to read music at sight – that is, to sing or play a composition you had never heard – but also to compose music "virtually" without performing it first.[3] The connection between the notes of a musical score and the relationships in sound they stood for had already become sufficiently natural by the early seventeenth century for Bacon to dismiss scholastic music theory and its preoccupation with numerical proportion as "reduced unto certain Mystical Subtleties, of no use, and not much Truth" (Bacon: 1628). In Bacon's lifetime, composers were more excited over the challenge of controlling the human spirit than establishing the structures controlling music.[4]

Early Modern Sound Studies

It is tempting to present the history of sound (or sound studies) and hearing's place in sensory culture as a newly emerging, or at least rapidly consolidating, branch of inquiry into the acoustic environment that many date back to the appearance of R. Murray Schafer's *The Soundscape: The Tuning of the World* (1977). A cluster of publications has recently appeared exploring the linkage between sound technologies and modern culture, notably Thompson's (2002) and Veit Erlmann's (2004) interdisciplinary volume. Mark M. Smith 2004 usefully historicizes this new work by anthologizing a series of writings defining the field since Schafer.[5] Smith's own introduction to what he calls the basics of historical acoustemology, auditory culture or aural history draws on the influential work of the anthropologist Steven Feld, who first coined the term "acoustemology" to denote the study of sound as a modality of knowing and being-in-the-world (Feld 1982).[6] Feld's acoustemology similarly frames *The Auditory Culture Reader*, a collection of new and previously published writings from anthropology, sociology, media studies, urban geography, philosophy, cultural studies and musicology which editors Michael Bull and Les Back want to be read as "a series of provocations towards *deep listening*" (Bull and Back 2003: 3).

Unsurprisingly, most of the literature referred to so far attends to sounds experienced in modern times, specifically since Thomas Edison announced his invention of the phonograph in 1877.[7] Indeed, it is this recording technology and its successive transformations through to the present digital age that fundamentally connect all sound-related academic research over the last four generations. The potential of sound technologies as tools *for* – as well as objects *of* – study continues to be explored right across the academy, in established research communities situated on each side of the sciences–humanities divide, in emerging disciplines that contest this division and in looser networks of scholars who traffic across domains. My essay explores some of the ways in which this global process has been played out locally in the early modern field, and has been framed as a personal response to an invitation I received to explore the range of recent work on the history of sound, particularly that of the early modern era from the perspective of intellectual history and the history of medicine and science.[8] I have organized my exploration along three pathways that have proved particularly fruitful for my own research into music's significance for early modern intellectual life, concentrating for the most part on English language sources by Anglo American trained scholars that relate to the period c. 1470–1740. As well as realizing how much has had to be left out, readers will also appreciate that my understanding of what is recent extends well before the 1990s. Nevertheless, I will begin by drawing attention to several monographs that have been published since then, to exemplify how sound history is currently being approached from different disciplines within the humanities (respectively English, Communications Studies, History and Religion): Smith 1999, Gouk 1999, Peters 1999 and Schmidt 2000.

In fact, there is a much larger body of relevant work on the early modern era by scholars who are not normally identified as historians of sound. Kahn 1999 is right to warn that musicology privileges a particularly Western sonic art. Nevertheless, it seems prudent for historians who want to integrate sound into their research to familiarize themselves with the methods that musicologists have been developing and the conceptual problems they have been addressing since the late nineteenth century in their study of musical sound.[9]

Early modernists who would like to "deepen their listening" have access to a wealth of scholarship exploring change and continuity in musical organization, both at the micro level of individual composers and their work, and at the macro level of particular periods and styles.[10] Perhaps more importantly for attempting deep listening, they also have access to a wealth of "early music" recordings and live performances, a vast body of audio and audiovisual material to which no electronic supplement I might offer here could do adequate justice.[11]

Of course, historians have always recognized music as a category worth considering, and there are excellent examples where it has been given a prominent place (for example, Hale 1971, especially Chapter 7, "The Arts and their Audience," and Burke 1978). However, whereas musicologists naturally turn to cultural studies for approaches that might help them to explain changes in music, historians do not routinely consider music itself as an agent or indicator of change. Compare this neglect to the way that visuality and techniques of picturing have become a vital part of the cultural historian's explanatory toolkit. Whatever the reality, it has become a truism that a reliance on vision at the expense of the other senses has come to make the "West" distinctively different from the "rest." (see, for example, Harvey 1990 and Crosby 1998). For Walter Ong (1958) and Marshall McLuhan (1962), the invention of the printing press signaled the beginning of Europe's first communications revolution, a new reproductive technology that Elizabeth Eisenstein (1979) further elaborated on as an agent of change in Western society. For Samuel Edgerton (1976), and more recently Martin Kemp (1990), the (re)discovery of linear perspective marked an equally critical turning-point in Western ways of knowing and understanding the world. And ever since Michael Baxandall first used the concept of the "period eye" in 1972 to talk about Renaissance painting, the cognitive skills shared by painters and the patronizing public and the value of these skills for Western intellectual life have become objects of debate (Baxandall 1972).

In contrast to an overwhelming fascination with visual technologies and power of the gaze, there has been comparatively little interest in the long-term cultural impact of new or "rediscovered" techniques for controlling musical sound that emerged in early modern Europe.[12] Despite equivalent advances in technologies of musical reproduction, the "period ear" and its cultural formation has only recently emerged as an explicit object of academic attention (Burstyn 1997). Whether aural technologies have as much power as visual technologies to alter physical and mental states, including the capacity to create new way of listening and thinking, is not yet recognized as a pressing historical question (Wegman 1998). However, I am confident that early modernists will become accustomed to using musical examples to help them think about changing soundscapes and aurality, just as they now use paintings and other images to think about landscapes and visuality. There is enormous potential for exploring how art music served as a powerful vehicle for organizing, controlling and giving meaning to early modern experience, an agent of cultural change but also continuity, a tool for negotiating relationships by subordinate as well as dominant groups.[13]

Indeed, it was precisely this potential for exercising control that fascinated Bacon, who in his *Sylva Sylvarum* (1627) laid out an investigative program for a new science of sound that already by the eighteenth century was becoming stabilized as "acoustics."[14] In Gouk (1999), which concentrates on the performative aspects of acoustics and the space it opened up between natural magic and the new, experimental philosophy, I emphasized Bacon's overlapping interests in "harmony" as instrumentally organized sound capable of altering bodily and mental states, and in "sympathy" or musical resonance as a model of occult action at a distance, a concept which Jamie Kassler (1995) shows was notably taken up by Hooke to explain mental functioning. What these studies did not bring out so clearly is the broader sensory framework in which these ideas were conceived, especially the connections between hearing and the other senses (inner as well as outer) that Bacon thought would be revealed if his ambitious plans for a comprehensive history of the senses – possibly the first initiative of this kind in history – were to be carried out.

Historians have been aware of the fundamentalist streak in Bacon's experimental agenda at least since Charles Webster (1974) drew attention to later English Baconian attempts to reform man's fallen nature, and their technologically-driven efforts to recreate a more authentic state. However, the centrality of sound to the Baconian goal of improving the human condition has scarcely begun to be explored, even though as Hillel Schwartz rightly observes, "sound was the environs through which Bacon intended to restore … the world to its proper senses" (Quoted with permission of Hillel Schwartz from a draft of his book-in-progress on the cultural history of noise, Round One [Chapter 2], to be published by Zone Books, New York.) This desire to improve or alter the state of humanity – or merely one's own state – through controlling and aligning sound has played a much greater part in European history than is generally appreciated. Fortunately, the task of reconnecting sound technology to statecraft is made easier once it is identified as part of the broader humanist agenda that has long been a fertile area for historical and philosophical debate.

Musical Humanism and Experimental Science

Two twentieth-century pioneers of early modern sound studies were D.P. Walker (1914–85), reader in Renaissance Studies at the University of London's Warburg Institute, and Claude Palisca (1921–2003), a Yale musicologist who specialized in the intellectual foundations of late Renaissance and Baroque music.[15] Beyond a shared enthusiasm for the art music of the period, what connected these scholars was an interest in "musical humanism," a term Walker coined around 1940 to signify the attempted reconstruction of ancient musical practices described in the Greek and Latin texts that were being studied the Italian Renaissance. Walker's interest was driven by a conviction that the ancient world really did provide humanists with "palpable models for music," just as it did for the plastic arts, even though musicologists of the 1920s and 1930s had assumed that there was no imitation of ancient music in the sixteenth century (Walker 1941–2: 1–13, 111–21, 220–7, 88–308, 55–71; Palisca 1985a). Walker, later followed by Palisca, proved conclusively that between the fifteenth and seventeenth centuries a number of so-called humanists (of various undefined occupational and social identities) began to formulate ideas about ancient music through close readings of Greek, Latin and even Hebrew texts, many of these becoming accessible in print for the first time. From this body of evidence they came to agree that ancient music was unlike modern music because it had astonishing power, one source of which was the proper union of music and poetry. If ancient wisdom were to be believed (for example, Plato, *Laws*, *Republic*), it was possible for special individuals to create certain kinds of organized sound or "harmony" that would improve personal and social well-being: specifically music that could be used to control strong passions, to inculcate virtue, to cure disease, and even to ensure the stability of the state (or to work the reverse).[16] On a less exalted plane, other ancient texts (for example, Vitruvius, Hero of Alexander) described ingenious musical marvels and acoustic wonders that delighted ancient emperors, technologies that again seemed to have no parallel in present times.[17]

On the page itself nothing appears particularly special about this information, because the "praise of music" was a literary tradition that went back many centuries (see, for example, Moyer 1992). Yet, from around the end of the fifteenth century, we have evidence that this body of data began to be interrogated more proactively, on the assumption that comparable transformations of the self and society might be achieved through appropriate technologies of sound. For although Walker did not mention the Florentine philosopher and priest Marsilio Ficino in his early articles on musical humanism, he later (Walker 1958: 1–24), certainly proves Ficino to have been engaged in a daring attempt to restore the lost sonic practices of Pythagoras and other ancient magi, an experimental endeavor that ostensibly relied on the natural properties of *spiritus* (a vital substance mediating between matter and intellect) for achieving therapeutic, if not explicitly theurgic, ends.[18]

Ficino seems to have been extreme in his imitation of pagan mysteries, but his approach to the past marks a new trend as early moderns increasingly began to reflect on the historical realities of ancient musical culture and its relevance to the present in ways that resonate with modern research questions: What did ancient music sound like and how was it made? What was the cause of music's power on individual and collective states in antiquity, and to what extent can this power be compared to that of modern music? What techniques would be required to reproduce these ancient effects authentically? These questions still remain challenging today, not only because the sounds of antiquity are forever lost, but also because the evidence that can be used to study them has not been added to significantly since the German Jesuit Athanasius Kircher published his comprehensive works on music, magic and acoustics during his career in Counter-Reformation Rome (see Gouk 2001: 71–83).[19]

This experimental trend, first documented in Medici Florence, was taken up in other courtly and civic contexts, notably when the need to restore or maintain harmony seemed particularly pressing. As the Reformation conflict fragmented Western Christendom, Protestants and Catholics alike looked to music as a force for reestablishing moral order, as well as recognizing its healing and restorative powers (see Ahmed 1997; Oettinger 2001). The earliest work to study in depth this linkage between idealized conceptions of ancient music and the resolution of modern discord through harmony was by Dame Frances Yates (1899–1981), a colleague of Walker's at the Warburg (Yates 1947: see especially, Chapters 3 and 4). Admittedly, Walker (1946–7) had already drawn attention to the revolutionary ambitions of Jean-Antoine de Baïf's Académie de Poésie et de Musique, but it was Yates who alerted scholars to the political and religious significance of Baïf's efforts to create a new kind of French song that followed the principles of ancient Greek verse. Baïf's academy – effectively the first state-funded research institute – was granted letters patent by Charles IX in 1570, in the throes of civil and religious conflict that threatened to destroy the French body politic, an action justified on the Platonic grounds that "the music current and used in the country should be retained under certain laws, for … where music is disordered, there morals are also depraved, and where it is well ordered, there men are well disciplined morally" (Yates 1947: App. 1 319–22). Yates's contribution to the debate on magic and the rise of modern science might seem outdated nowadays, but her insights in this book about the connections between new music, new academies and the "new science," framed within the demands of political survival are worth revisiting. More clearly than Walker or Palisca, she showed the power of early modern philosophers to change the nature of music, and that music itself had the power to change philosophers' minds (through the use of musical models for understanding the world).[20]

Over the last half century, this mutual cognitive and cultural transformation has not been studied as a single phenomenon effected through sound. Instead it has been fragmented across several academic fields that share interests in the High Renaissance and its patronage of sciences and the arts (see Shirley and Hoeniger

1985). Thus, some of the consequences of the desire to recreate particular effects achieved in antiquity are familiar to musicologists in the context of a revolution in *musical* practice that took place around 1600. It was Palisca (1960) who showed how the new Baroque style of monody (flexible solo song with chordal accompaniment) and opera emerged out of attempts to restore the ancient Greek ideal of expressing the "affect" or emotional character of the words being set to music (see also Katz 1984: 361–77). Now, for the first time, composers were declaring their intention to express the passions of the soul, and to move the affections of their audiences. The origins of this new trend can be traced to the Florentine Camerata, a group of musical amateurs who met at Count Giovanni Bardi's house in the 1570s and 80s. A leading figure in this movement was Vincenzo Galilei, father of Galileo and Michelagnolo, of whom only the latter went on make a living through music, although both brothers were skilled lutenists like their father (see Drake 1970a: 43–62; Palisca 1985a: 265–79).

The Galileo connection immediately suggests why other evidence of this sonic transformation is familiar to historians of science, in the context of an early modern revolution in *scientific* practice: a paradigm shift embodied in the instrumentally- and also mathematically-based method of generating understanding about the world that established Galileo's position as philosopher to the Medici Grand Duke of Tuscany in 1610. This convergence between the musical, mathematical and scientific in one of the icons of the Scientific Revolution (and indeed several other icons, notably Kepler, Descartes, Mersenne, Huygens and Euler) has naturally attracted attention from scholars other than Palisca and Walker.[21] Foremost among their generation were Stillman Drake (1914–93), Alistair Crombie (1915–96) and Clifford Truesdell (1919–2000).[22] Those still living whose research has most obviously centered on and sustained this theme of harmonics, or what we might call "music as history of early modern science," include H. Floris Cohen, Sigalia Dostrovsky, Paolo Gozza, Jamie C. Kassler and the author.[23] To this core can be added contributions by Albert Cohen (1981; and, with Leta Miller, 1987), Thomas Christensen (1993) and Victor Coelho (1992).

All are recommended reading for early modern sound studies, but, in this limited space, I will concentrate on what Cohen (1984: 1–12) first identified as the "problem of consonance" and its drastic redefinition by theorists between around 1580 and 1650. This problem was directly related to the transition from two- to three-dimensional pitch space (analogous to the shift to linear perspective already described). Before this period, theories of harmony were confined to musical sounds heard melodically (as, for example, in church modes) and consonance was defined through the ratios of the Pythagorean scale. By 1650 an alternative way of conceptualizing harmony had emerged, a tonal system where musical intervals are heard simultaneously (that is to say, harmonically). The scale itself became the subject of disagreement, because the Pythagorean system did not allow thirds and sixths to be harmonic intervals, even though they were clearly being composed and heard as though they were. (For an introduction to this complex field see Rasch 2002 and Gouk 2002: 193–222, 223–45.) In *Quantifying Music* (1984) Floris Cohen explores the mathematical, experimental and mechanistic methods his "scientists" developed to analyze the shifting grounds of consonance, practices that appear coextensive with the emergence of modern physical science. Kassler (1995) extends this story with English "philosophers" grappling with consonance into the eighteenth century, her first case being Hobbes (who, like Galileo, was also a lutenist) in his influential *Human Nature* (1650). These studies indicate there was a transformation in the nature of musical experience itself, as the soundscape of composed art music was itself transformed.

Performance Practice and the Early Music Movement

Yet, even as consonance is fruitfully brought to the foreground in these studies, what remains as background are the sounds, the instruments, the performers and the specific aural/social contexts which made music perception become a subject of learned discourse in the first place. In my experience, an effective way of connecting studies in the history of early modern science to early music history is by concentrating on performance practice, and its implications for the formation of social and personal identities (see Gouk 1996; 2005; for music and identity formation in a later period see Leppert 1993). The changes in musical experience (for example, the sounds "themselves" being judged as consonant or not) that led to a reconceptualization of musical space and time were associated with specific instrumental and vocal practices that became established in late fifteenth- and sixteenth-century Europe. Both the source of, and the solutions to, the problem of consonance prove to be located in the growing use of certain instruments (for example, keyboards, lutes, viols) during this period, especially for accompanying verse (see Wainwright and Holman 2005; for further information on specific instruments see Sadie 1984]).

Emmanuel Winternitz (1982; 1979), for example, drew attention to the convergence of musical and visual imagination in Leonardo's inventions, while Stillman Drake (1975: 98–104; 1970) highlighted the importance of Galileo's lute training for his experiments measuring the speed of falling bodies, practices which relied on an internalized ability to keep regular time. Drake could equally well have stressed the importance to any lutenist of keeping in tune, an ongoing process of adjusting string tension, the position of the frets on the fingerboard and the placing of the fingers themselves, all this coordination being more difficult in consort than in solo settings. Similar observations can be made about the technical demands placed on keyboard players, and the modifications they made before and during performance – for example, transposition (to match voice range) as well as temperament (to play chords in tune) (see Lindley 1984; 2001: 248–68). What this adds up to is that professional musicians were grappling empirically with the consequences of new musical technologies long before they caught the attention of Cohen's "scientists," a category of intellectuals whose members became conversant with such problems in social contexts where musical literacy was desirable and expected.

This should remind us that a primary function of music making was to negotiate social relationships, and that fashions in music as well as behavior were set among intellectual elites. Harmony, in other words (that is, as music actually played and sung by courtiers, as well as danced to or listened to), should be added to the control mechanisms that Stephen Greenblatt (1980) and Mario Biagioli (1992) have identified as essential to the construction of courtly behavior and modes of critical, even "scientific" perception. Although not all aristocrats created music (most just relied on professionals to do this for them), in contexts where high-ranking patrons cultivated skills of performance the techniques they used naturally became indicators of gentility and high intellect. Thus when Lorenzo de' Medici sang lyrics to his own accompaniment, for example, this became an intrinsically noble practice (see D'Accone 1993: 229–48). Jeanice Brooks (2000) shows this "Medici" phenomenon at work in the Valois court, a body that defined itself through the performance of *airs de cour* which created a sense of belonging and place.[24]

The extensive resources now available for historians wishing to acquaint themselves with a genre like the *air de cour* or any other form of early music stem from a movement that became professionalized in the 1970s, although having much older roots (see Weber 1992). At first the term "early music" was limited to music of the Baroque and earlier periods (which is to say before 1750), but has since become used to denote "any music for which a historically appropriate style of performance must be reconstructed" (Haskell 2001: 831–4 at 831). What I find interesting is the resemblance between this movement as it has developed since the late nineteenth century, and the Renaissance humanist project that Walker uncovered, in that both appear to have been driven by a desire for radical authenticity, the recreation of a lost art through appropriate interrogation of historical data (see Tomlinson 1998: 115–36). Just as Palisca showed was the case for Vincenzo Galilei and his collaborators, so present reconstruction of past musical practices relies on philological examination of surviving scores, treatises and other textual evidence, as well as studies of instruments and other artifacts, and results have to be tested and demonstrated experimentally.

The only major difference between the Camerata's experiments and those of more recent early-music enthusiasts seems to be improved sound recording technology – for example, the launch of LPs in 1948 being identified in the twenty-fifth anniversary issue of

Early Music (1997) as a crucial factor in its own success.[25] Other journals that chart developments in this significant area of early modern sound studies include the more academically-oriented *Early Music History* (1981) and the *Galpin Society Journal* launched in 1946 to commemorate the pioneering work of Canon F. W. Galpin (1858–1945) on the history, construction, development and use of musical instruments. A recent trend in early music scholarship has been towards the listeners' experience of performance, a deliberate shift away from the technologies of production towards consumption that parallels earlier moves in history of medicine to the "patients' point of view" (see, for example, Porter 1985). There has also been more conscious focus on urban soundscapes, and the integration of music into the architecture of power (see Burgess and Wathey 2000: 1-46; Kisby 2001: 1–13).

However, there is still work to be done integrating urban studies with the excellent literature now available on the manufacture, maintenance and circulation of instruments as evidence of soundscape control, such as Lindley (1984), Woodfield (1988) and O'Brien (1990). To complement these studies of music technology that were defining inner, domestic space, Polk (1992), Barclay (1992) and Waterhouse (1994) uncover the world of ceremonial, public music, which, due to its mostly outdoor nature, was dominated by brass and wind. In the surviving repertory of written music there is scant record of the communities of artisans who made and played these instruments, their activities supported by imperial cities, towns and every significant institution willing to pay for these aural manifestations of "stature, stability and power" (Polk 1992: 3). Unsurprisingly, the epicenters of manufacture (notably in German-speaking lands) prove to be precisely those generating the practitioners whose skills in crafting precision instruments and natural knowledge have long been preoccupying historians and curators of scientific instruments – a community whose desire to preserve and bring to life old instruments clearly overlaps with that of the early-music movement. In the 1964 volume of *Technology and Culture* Derek de Solla Price and Silvio Bedini were already drawing attention to early automata and their relationship to the mechanical philosophy (de Solla Price 1964; Bedini 1964;more recently the essays in Moran 1991b). The extent of the convergence between musical and mathematical control, and their impact on the sonic environment, can also be gleaned from books such as those by Maurice and Mayer (1980) and Haspels (1987).

Harmony as Healing: Restoring Spirits and Uplifting Souls

In this final section, I want to turn my attention from sonic acts of imaginative reconstruction designed to connect their performers to a more authentic past and towards musical technologies of healing that occupy the contested domain of performing cures. If we think about these apparently very different applications of sound control in terms of the Baconian quest for human perfectibility, the boundaries between "music" and "medicine" are blurred: through sound alignment it may prove possible to restore balance within individual human and also social bodies, to maintain harmony between inner self and outer cosmos: in short, to achieve a better state. Such goals were certainly being pursued during the sixteenth-century religious wars; Yates (1947) for example, shows that Charles IX supported Baïf's institutionalized attempts to create a powerful new kind of song because it might restore health to the ailing body politic. This was called *musique mesurée à l'antique*, a form in which French words were set to music according to the principles used in Greek measured verse, with a view to creating the same kind of ethical effects that were described in antiquity (Walker and Lesure [1949: 151–70]). Ironically, the same humanist ideals underpinned the songs that the king (and most of his Catholic supporters) identified as a principal cause of social malaise: the psalms and hymns through which the Huguenots maintained their religious identity and attracted new converts to the Protestant cause (see Diefendorf 1993: 41–63). The quest to realign divine and human music also had implications for personal health; from Walker (1958: 96–106) we learn that it was also in 1570s Paris that Jacques Gohory, one of the first authors to introduce Paracelsian medicine into France, established a private academy where he experimented with amulets intended to harness the natural influence of the stars – an operation that Ficino argued in his *De Vita* was best achieved through imitating the Orphic rites. A similar dedication to the pursuit of spiritual medicines in the face of deepening crisis is found a few decades later in the Kassel court of Moritz of Hessen, who was an accomplished musician and poet as well as the foremost patron of the occult philosophy in Europe (see Moran 1991a). Kassel became a magnet for a wide spectrum of mystical philosophers and alchemists as Moritz turned from his failing public life towards a magically-based experimental philosophy that would provide effective salves for individual and political health (also compare Evans 1973). Occult philosophers were confident that "Musicall harmony" empowered the pious practitioner to achieve wondrous effects (as in the 1651 English translation of H.C. Agrippa's *Three Books of Occult Philosophy*, Book II, cap.8 [Agrippa 1986]). Thus, the earliest image of an experimental laboratory spells out that "Sacred music is the escape from sadness and evil spirits because the spirit (*spiritus*) rejoices cheerfully in a heart filled with pious joy."[26] Through his desire to harness the harmonies governing nature for the relief of physical and mental suffering, the magus is identified with King David, the charismatic leader of the Israelites who, according to the Old Testament, was inspired by the Holy Spirit to sing God's praises through voice and harp. In the seventeenth century not just court physicians, but anyone versed in Scripture knew that psalmody was a means of raising spirits and restoring souls, just as they knew that David's ability to cure Saul's mental anguish and gift of prophecy came through the wondrous power of song (see Gouk 2005).

According to one of the main narrative threads of Western intellectual history, the occult belief in the macrocosm–microcosm analogy became obsolete by the eighteenth century. The Enlightenment myth that scientific rationalism gradually displaced religious and magical beliefs is slowly being discredited, but some analytical frameworks still wielded by historians of medicine (and also of music) – including the development of a more objectifying, visualist culture at the expense of the other senses – presume there was a process of "disenchantment" taking place from the late seventeenth century, one which meant that music, society and the cosmos were no longer held together, and the harmony of the spheres fell silent (for example, James [1993]). Whether this actually happened or not is difficult to find out, because since music and cosmology now seem so obviously distinct from each other there appears to be no common interest among historians in trying to explain how they might actually be connected in the modern world, or how such connections might be mediated through the embodied, sensory experience of what might be naively described as "music itself."

I only began to realize the limiting effect of this "non-question," or absence of anything to explain, about a decade ago when I embarked on a project exploring the relationship between music and healing in Western society since the Renaissance. Conscious of knowing practically nothing about comparative systems of healing outside the Western paradigm, and reluctant to take "music" and "medicine" as self-evident categories, I convened an interdisciplinary symposium as part of the Sixteenth Congress of the International Musicological Society in 1997, the fruits of which appeared in Gouk (2000).[27] As hoped for, the editor learned a great deal from her contributors (and their reading lists), several of whom also wrote complementary essays for Horden, 2000 (see, for example, Austern 2000b 213–45; Kramer 2000a 338–52). This finally brings me to the last group of texts that I want to recommend for early modern sound studies, a genre already mentioned in the context of Steven Feld's influential recordings of rainforest music and their implications for theorizing a culture's embodied sense of place.

Acoustemology has deservedly gained attention from outside anthropology, but, among practitioners themselves, Feld's approach is not exceptional. Back in 1973, when early-music and folk enthusiasts were also signaling fresh directions for musicology, John Blacking (1928–90) was probably right to assert that ethnomusicology's new method of analyzing music and music history based on the assumption "that because music is humanly organized sound, there ought to be a relationship between patterns of human organization and patterns of sound produced as human interaction" commanded little respect (Blacking 1976: 26). Since then, however, Blacking's claim that "music" functions as a primary modeling system in non-Western societies has gained increasing authority, as has the basic ethnographic premise that to discover the meanings of the institutions and practices in a given culture these have to be mapped on to that culture's larger world view. Thus, at a conference in 2002, for example, Anthony Seeger explained that his (1987) investigation *Why Suyá Sing* was driven by the desire to "understand the relationship between ways that people conceive of their universe (cosmology), organize themselves into groups (social organization) and organize sounds (music and some of the features of language)" (Seeger 2002). And as I was grateful to acknowledge in my introduction to *Musical Healing*, other notable studies that explore the connection between musical and health care systems include Janzen (1991), Roseman (1991) and Friedson (1996). Just as the editors of *The Auditory Culture Reader* recommend, these authors sought to overcome the preconceptions embedded in a visualist metaphysics and instead tried to *listen to* what healing entails, to imagine a reality where "music" is not subordinate or peripheral to some other kind of process, but is the activity which (in the case of Friedson's dancing prophets, for example) at once constitutes the disease and the diagnosis.

Comparable work on a European theme being undertaken around this time included Cheryce Kramer's (1998) investigation of a nineteenth-century asylum at Illenau, near Dresden. Kramer's contribution to *Musical Healing* reflects on her finding that pre-Freudian German psychiatry was directed towards a peculiar soul-organ called the *Gemüth*, a collectively instantiated entity which "suffered its own forms of illness ... and was particularly susceptible to sensory stimulation, especially music" (2000a: 137–48, qtn 138). In the conclusion to her chapter she argues for a linkage between the musical therapeutics practiced at Illenau, the example of "doing ngoma" seen in 1982 in Greater Capetown by Janzen, and the musical performances marking the transition from sickness to health Henry Stobart witnessed during his 1990s fieldwork in a remote hamlet in the Bolivian Andes (Stobart 2000: 26–45). According to Kramer, these very different musical events appear quite similar "if we focus not on the content of individual healing rituals but on their cultural function," a possibly defining feature of music therapy being the affinity between particular soul types such as *animu*, "spirits" and *Gemüth*, and particular musical cures, that is to say, "music congruent with the configuration of soul deemed most restorative at a given time and place" (2000b: 146).

It may still be too soon to evaluate Kramer's hypothesis, but to my mind one striking piece of evidence that supports her functionalist approach is *Music and Medicine* (Schullian and Schoen 1948). At the time of its publication Schullian was a librarian in the history section of the Army Services Medical Library (later the National Library of Medicine), while Schoen was the Head of Education and Psychology at the Carnegie Institute of Technology. As Schullian

(1948: 407–71) knew from her historical survey of literature on music and medicine, this was the first coordinated attempt to address the scientific and historical aspects of music therapy. Indeed, *Music and Medicine* itself provided the academic legitimacy for music therapy becoming a fully accredited profession in the United States. Much can be learned from this assemblage of writings by a diverse group of professionals, whom the editors recognized as having authority to speak on music and medicine in past, present and future states.[28] In the context of sound studies, what fascinates me most is Schullian's account of the tangled motives she thought lay behind the volume, which was apparently first conceived of in 1944 by the Officer-in-Charge of the US Army Medical Library. First, Schullian observes that "the tragic years of World War II witnessed a dramatic growth in the interdependence of music and medicine," a growth which she saw manifested in "the heightened role played by music therapy in military hospitals." On the one hand, this scholarly initiative was symptomatic of a more general desire to restore harmony that gained momentum during the war effort. Nationwide "musicians by the hundreds … sought entrance to the hospitals to bring with their music comfort to the men and women who had become incapacitated in the service of their country" (Van de Wall 1948: 293–321 at 294), on the other, as Schullian goes on to admit, it proved impossible to harmonize "the complicated forces acting upon one another in the fields of music and medicine, and the result in too many cases was confusion and bewilderment" Thus, the exceptional wartime events that instigated a concerted move to relieve suffering also led to discord between individuals whose interests overlapped on the borders of existing, redefining and newly emerging disciplines in the struggle to control the place of music in hospitals and other medical institutions.

Music and the Paradox of Power

Writing at the dawn of a new century, Francis Bacon had a profound conviction that his motivations for, and methods of, creating sound history were novel and powerful. Conscious of new and exciting musical technologies that were dazzling everyone around him, he dismissed established methods of recording sounds without realizing how fundamental these structures were to his own powers of thought. We are also living in an age of new and rapidly developing technologies that promise to improve our scholarship, so that, since the 1970s, sound studies and sensory history have offered ever-growing opportunities for making deeper and more integrated connections with the past, of recovering alternative modes of being and subaltern states. While demonstrating commitment to this ideal, we should not underestimate the capacity to forget earlier projects which had similar designs in mind. In the 1940s, as we have seen, a small group of classically-trained scholars were already discovering evidence of Renaissance projects to change the state of the world through sound, an indication that the roots of sound history may be as old as writing history itself. In conjunction with more recent studies (notably in the history of science, in early music history and ethnomusicology), I have drawn attention to some early modern experiments to use music as an agent of change, examples of sound control that include (a) attempts to recover a more authentic song, conducted in the hope of restoring connection to a lost but golden past, or of bringing back a proper community spirit; (b) attempts to restore harmony in a chaotic world, the reintegration of a universe that is fragmented and out of joint; and (c) attempts to find cures for troubled spirits, medicines that will heal soul sickness and restore inner peace. The paradox is that even as we may celebrate sound studies, resistance to the power of music is still institutionally maintained – hence my experience of the difficulty of reintegrating music into the fabric of intellectual and cultural history, of the resistance to granting music a central role in philosophical and scientific change, and the reluctance to accede to ancient (and popular) notions of its redemptive and restorative powers.

Acknowledgments

Thanks are due to Hillel Schwartz and Anthony Grafton, Jeffrey Dean and Tom Dixon for their reading of an earlier draft of this article.

Notes

1. Lindsay 1911, I: K6^r. Although Isidore did not know it, by the fourth century BC the Greeks had already developed two parallel systems of notation, one used for vocal, the other for instrumental, music, see West 1992: 7.
2. For an introduction see Apel (1953), Rastall (1983) and Tanay (1999).
3. Lydia Goehr (1992) argues that the concept of a musical work emerged around 1800. However, the writings of the music theorist Johannes Tinctoris in the 1470s, naming individual compositions and their composers, and criticizing their faults and virtues, demonstrate a sufficiently strong work-concept (if not so absolute as that treated by Goehr) to have been operative in the fifteenth century (Tinctoris 1975–6). For a list of English translations of Tinctoris' works see, Ronald Woodley's "Johannes Tinctoris" in *New Grove* (2001) 25: 500–1.
4. Bacon's interest in music's power over the spirit was first explored by D.P. Walker (1972: 121–30).
5. For the period before 1700 Smith 2004 includes abridged versions of Burnett (1991: 43–69); Gouk (1991: 95–113) and Woolf (1986: 159–93).
6. As a documentary sound artist Feld has also produced recordings like *Bosavi: Rainforest Music from Papua New Guinea* (Smithsonian Folkways Recordings, CD 40487, 2001) and *Bells and Winter Festivals of Greek Macedonia* (Smithsonian Folkways CD 50401, 2002).

7. In addition to works cited above and in Smith's essay see, for example, Bijsterveld and Pinch (2004), and Alter and Koepnick (2004).
8. Mark Smith, personal communication.
9. I use the term "musicology" in the widest sense to include ethnomusicology and related fields; for an overview see Duckles et. al. (2001: 488–533).
10. See, for example, *Journal of the Royal Musical Association*, *Journal of the American Musicological Association*, *Music & Letters*, *Early Music History*, *Early Music*, *Revue de musicologie*.
11. One point of entry into this material being, for example, http://www.earlymusic.net/home.html (accessed 22.10.05).
12. An early exception to this rule being Lowinsky (1946). Two more recent works (both translations from the French), that challenge, but hardly disprove my claim, are Attali (1985) and Poizat (1992).
13. For musicology's limitations and strengths as a tool for the social analysis of sound, see Shepherd, *Music as Social Text* (1991).
14. Joseph Sauveur (1653–1715) thought he was the first to coin the term *l'acoustique*, as in his *Collected Writings on Musical Acoustics*, (Rasch 1984), but it is clear that "acoustics" was being used in England much earlier; see Chapter 5 of Gouk 1999.
15. On Palisca see Paula Morgan, "Claude Palisca" in *New Grove* (2001) 19: 3–5; for Walker see the bibliography in Walker (1985: 1–5) and Penelope Gouk *New Grove* (2001) 27: 29.
16. For an introduction to the Greek sources (of which only a handful was still unknown to scholars by 1500) see Barker (1984; 1989). On equivalent Hebrew sources see Shiloah (1993). For a survey of ancient literate traditions on music's therapeutic power (Chinese, Greek, Indian, Jewish and Muslim) see the essays in Horden (2000).
17. This material has been studied in the context of Renaissance theater and garden design rather than from the perspective of humanism; see, for example, Yates (1969) and Strong (1979).
18. For later interpretations of Ficino's experiments see Godwin (1987: 24–5 esp.); Tomlinson (1993: 101–44); Voss (2002: 227–42); Gouk (2004: 87–105).
19. For comparable modern reflections on such problems see Kenyon (1988) and Buckley (1998).
20. For a general introduction to musical models see Kassler (1982).
21. But see first, Palisca (1961: 91–137; 1985b: 59–73) and D.P. Walker (1978: 14–26, 27–33, 34–62).
22. Drake (1970b: 483–500; 1970a: 43–62); Crombie (1990a: 93–117; 1990b: "Mathematics, Music and Medical Science,"

363-378; 1971: 295–309); Truesdell (1960: 15–141; 1955: xix–xxiv).
23. Cohen (1984); Dostrovsky (1974–5: 169–218); Cannon and Dostrovsky (1981); Gozza (1989; 2000); Kassler (1979; 1995; 2001); Gouk (1999).
24. Brooks uses the prefatory material in Adrien le Roy's 1571 *Livre d'airs de cour miz sur le luth* as a guide to the courtly identities constructed through song. On the dance and courtly self-presentation see McGowan (1963) and McClary (1998: 85–112).
25. This special issue was devoted to listening practice.
26. Heinrich Khunrath's self-portrait in his *Amphitheatrum sapientiae aeternae* (1st edn 1595, 2nd edn 1609). For an online image and discussion see http://www.library.wisc.edu/libraries/SpecialCollections/khunrath/ (accessed October 22, 2005).
27. Chapters in Gouk 2000 relevant to this essay but not cited elsewhere include Burnett 2000 (85–91); Rousseau 2000 (92–112); Austern 2000a (113–36).
28. For further details, see Gouk 2000 (171–96). Most of the contributions had already appeared in academic books and journals, including *Musical Quarterly*, *Educational Music Magazine*, *Journal of Nervous and Mental Diseases*, and *American Journal of Psychiatry*.

References

Agrippa, H.C. 1986. *Three Books of Occult Philosophy*. 2nd edn. Facsimile. London: Chthonios Books.

Ahmed, Ehsan. 1997. *The Law and the Song: Hebraic, Christian and Pagan Revivals in Sixteenth-Century France*. Birmingham, AL: Summa publications.

Alter, Nora M. and Koepnick, Lutz (eds). 2004. *Sound Matters: Essays on the Acoustics of German Culture*. New York: Berghahn Books.

Apel, W. 1953. *The Notation of Polyphonic Music 900–1600*. 5th edn. Cambridge, MA: Mediaeval Academy of America.

Attali, Jacques. 1985. *Noise: The Political Economy of Music*. Trans. Brian Massumi. Minneapolis: University of Minnesota Press.

Austern, Linda Phyllis. 2000a. "'No Pill's Gonna Cure My Ill': Gender, Erotic Melancholy and Traditions of Musical Healing in the Modern West." In P. Gouk, *Musical Healing in Cultural Contexts*. Aldershot: Ashgate.

——. 2000b. "Musical Treatments for Lovesickness: The Early Modern Heritage." In Peregrine Horden (ed.), *Music as Medicine: The History of Music Therapy since Antiquity*. Aldershot: Ashgate.

Bacon, Francis. 1628. *Sylva Sylvarum: or a Naturall Historie. In Ten Centuries ... Published after the Authors death by William Rawley*. London: printed by J. H[aviland and A. Mathewes] for William Lee at the Turkes Head in Fleet-street, next to the Miter, § 101.

Barclay, Robert. 1992. *Art of the Trumpet-Maker: The Materials, Tools, and Techniques of the Seventeenth and Eighteenth Centuries in Nuremberg*. Oxford: Oxford University Press.

Barker, Andrew (ed.) 1984. *Greek Musical Writings, Vol. 1: The Musician and his Art*. Cambridge: Cambridge University Press.

——. (ed.) 1989. *Greek Musical Writings, Vol. 2: Harmonic and Acoustic Theory*. Cambridge: Cambridge University Press.

Baxandall, Michael. 1972. "The Period Eye." *Painting and Experience in Fifteenth-Century Italy*. Oxford: Oxford University Press.

Bedini, Silvio A. 1964. "The Role of Automata in the History of Technology." *Technology and Culture* 5: 24–42.

Biagioli, Mario. 1992. *Galileo, Courtier*. Chicago: University of Chicago Press.

Bijsterveld, Karin and Pinch, Trevor. 2004. "Sound Studies: New Technologies and Music." In *Social Studies of Science*, 34.

Brooks, Jeanice. 2000. *Courtly Song in Late Sixteenth-Century France*. Chicago: University of Chicago Press.

Buckley, Ann (ed.). 1998. *Hearing the Past: Essays in Historical Ethnomusicology and the Archaeology of Sound*. Liège: Université de Liège.

Bull, Michael and Back, Les. 2003. *The Auditory Culture Reader*. Oxford and New York: Berg.

Burgess, Clive and Wathey, Andrew. 2000. "Mapping the Soundscape: Church Music in English Towns, 1450–1550." *Early Music History*, 19: 1–46.

Burke, Peter. 1978. *Popular Culture in Early Modern Europe*. London: Temple Smith.

Burnett, Charles. 1991. "Sound and Its Perception in the Middle Ages." In Charles Burnett, Michael Fend and Penelope Gouk (eds), *The Second Sense: Studies in Hearing and Musical Judgement from Antiquity to the Seventeenth Century*. London: Warburg Institute.

Burnett, Charles. 2000. "'Spiritual Medicine': Music and Healing in Islam and its Influence in Western Medicine." In P. Gouk (ed.), *Musical Healing in Cultural Contexts*. Aldershot: Ashgate.

Burstyn, Shai. 1997. "In Quest of the Period Ear." *Early Music*, 25 (4): 692–702.

Cannon, J.T. and Dostrovsky, Sigalia. 1981. *The Evolution of Dynamics: Vibration Theory from 1687 to 1742*. New York: Springer-Verlag.

Christensen, Thomas. 1993. *Rameau and Musical Thought in the Enlightenment*. Cambridge: Cambridge University Press.

Coelho, Victor (ed.).1992. *Music and Science in the Age of Galileo*. Dordrecht: Kluwer.

Cohen, Albert. 1981. *Music in the French Royal Academy of Sciences: A Study in the Evolution of Musical Thought*. Princeton: Princeton University Press.

Cohen, H. Floris. 1984. *Quantifying Music: The Science of Music at the First Stage of the Scientific Revolution, 1580–1650*. Dordrecht: D. Reidel.

Crombie, Alistair C. 1990. "The Study of the Senses in Renaissance Science." In *Science, Optics and Music in Medieval and Early Modern Thought*. London: Hambledon Press.

———. 1990b. "Mathematics, Music and Medical Science." *Science, Optics and Music in Medieval and Early Modern Thought*. London: Hambledon Press.

Crosby, Alfred W. 1998: *The Measure of Reality: Quantification and Western Society 1250–1600*. Cambridge: Cambridge University Press.

D'Accone, Frank A.D. 1993. "Lorenzo il Magnifico e la musica." In Piero Gargiulo (ed.), *La musica a Firenze al tempo di Lorenzo il Magnifico*. Florence: Olschki.

de Solla Price, Derek J. 1964. "Automata in History. Automata and the Origins of Mechanism and Mechanistic Philosophy." *Technology and Culture*, 5: 9–23.

Diefendorf, Barbara B. 1993. "The Huguenot Psalter and the Faith of French Protestants in the Sixteenth Century.' In Barbara B. Diefendorf and C. Hesse (eds), *Culture and Identity in Early Modern Europe (1500–1800)*. Ann Arbor, MI: University of Michigan Press.

Dostrovsky, Sigalia. 1974–5. "Early Vibration Theory: Physics and Music in the Seventeenth Century." *Archive for the History of Exact Sciences*, 14: 169–218.

Drake, Stillman. 1970a. "Vincenzo Galilei and Galileo" In S. Drake (ed.), *Galileo Studies: Personality, Tradition and Revolution*. Michigan: Ann Arbor.

———. 1970b. "Renaissance Music and Experimental Science." *Journal of the History of Ideas*, 31: 483–500.

———. 1975. "The Role of Music in Galileo's Experiments." *Scientific American*, (Jan–June): 98–104.

Duckles et. al. 2001. "Musicology." In Stanely Sadie (ed.), *The New Grove Dictionary of Music and Musicians*, Vol. 17. 2nd edn. London: Macmillan.

Egerton, jr, Samuel Y. 1976. *The Renaissance Rediscovery of Linear Perspective*. New York: Harper Row.

Eisenstein, Elizabeth L. 1979. *The Printing Press as an Agent of Change*. Cambridge: Cambridge University Press.

Erlmann, Veit. 2004. *Hearing Cultures: Essays on Sound, Listening and Modernity*. Oxford and New York: Berg.

Evans, Rudolf. 1973. *Rudolf II and His World: A Study in Intellectual History 1576–1612*. Oxford: Oxford University Press.

Feld, Steven. 1982. *Sound and Sentiment: Birds, Weeping, Poetics, and Song in Kaluli Expression*. Philadelphia: University of Pennsylvania Press.

Feld, Steven and Basso, Keith H. (eds). 1996. *Senses of Place*. Santa Fe, NM: School of American Research Press ; [Seattle] : Distributed by the University of Washington Press

Freedman, Richard. 2000. *The Chansons of Orlando Di Lasso and Their Protestant Listeners: Music, Piety and Print in Sixteenth-Century France*. Rochester, NY: University of Rochester Press.

Friedson, Steven. 1996. *Dancing Prophets: Musical Experience in Tumbuka Healing*. Chicago and London: University of Chicago Press.

Godwin, Joscelyn. 1987. *Harmonies of Heaven and Earth: The Spiritual Dimension of Music from Antiquity to the Avant-Garde*. London: Thames and Hudson.

Goehr, Lydia. 1992. *The Imaginary Museum of Musical Works: An Essay in the Philosophy of Music*. Oxford: Clarendon Press.

Gouk, Penelope. 1991. "Some English Theories of Hearing in the Seventeenth Century: Before and after Descartes." In C. Burnett, M. Fend and P. Gouk (eds), *The Second Sense*. London: The Warburg Institute.

——. 1996. "Performance Practice: Music, Medicine and Natural Philosophy in Interregnum Oxford." *British Journal for the History of Science*, 29: 257–88.

——. 1999. *Music, Science and Natural Magic in Seventeenth-Century England*. New Haven and London: Yale University Press.

——. (ed.). 2000. *Musical Healing in Cultural Contexts*. Aldershot: Ashgate.

——. 2001. "Making Music, Making Knowledge: The Harmonious Universe of Athanasius Kircher." In Daniel Stolzenberg (ed.), *The Great Art of Knowing: The Baroque Encyclopaedia of Athanasius Kircher*. Standford: Stanford University Libraries.

——. 2002. "The Role of Harmonics in the Scientific Revolution." In Thomas Christensen (ed.), *The Cambridge History of Western Music Theory*. Cambridge: Cambridge University Press.

——. 2004 "Raising Spirits and Restoring Souls: Early Modern Medical Explanations for Music's Effects." In Veit Erlmann (ed.), *Hearing Cultures: Essays on Sound, Listening and Modernity* Berg, Oxford and New York.

——. 2005. "Harmony, Health and Healing: Music's Role in Early Modern Paracelsian Thought." In Margaret Pelling and Scott Mandelbrote (eds), *The Practice of Reform in Health, Medicine and Science, 1500–2000: Essays for Charles Webster*. Aldershot: Ashgate.

Gozza, Paolo (ed.). 1989. *La musica nella rivoluzione scientifica del seicento*. Bologna: Il Mulino.

——. (ed.). 2000. *Number to Sound: The Musical Way to the Scientific Revolution*. Dordrecht: Kluwer.

Greenblatt, Stephen. 1980. *Renaissance Self-Fashioning*. Chicago: University of Chicago Press.

Hale, John R. 1971. *Renaissance Europe: The Individual and Society, 1480–1520*. London: Fontana.

Harvey, David. 1990. *The Condition of Postmodernity: An Enquiry into the Origins of Cultural Change*. Cambridge, MA: Basil Blackwell Ltd, Cambridge, MA & Oxford.

Haskell, Harry. 2001. "Early music." In Stanely Sadie (ed.), *The New Grove Dictionary of Music and Musician*s, Vol. 7, 2nd edn. London: Macmillan.

Haspels, Jan Jaap. 1987. *Automatic Musical Instruments: Their Mechanics and Their Music 1580–1820*. Koedijk: Nirota, Muziekdruk C.V.

Horden, Peregrine (ed.). 2000. *Music as Medicine: The History of Music Therapy since Antiquity.* Part One. Aldershot: Ashgate.

James, Jamie. 1993. *The Music of the Spheres: Music, Science and the Natural Order of the Universe*. London: Little, Brown and Company.

Janzen, John. 1991. *Ngoma: Discourses of Healing in Central and Southern Africa*. Berkeley: University of California Press.

Kahn, Douglas. 1999. *Noise Water Meat: A History of Sound in the Arts*. Cambridge, MA: MIT Press.

Kassler, Jamie Croy. 1979. *The Science of Music in Britain 1714–1830: A Catalogue of Writings, Lectures and Inventions*. 2 vols. New York and London: Garland.

———. 1982. "Music as a Model in Early Science." *History of Science* xx: 103–39.

———. 1995. *Inner Music: Hobbes, Hooke and North on Internal Character*. London: Athlone Press.

———. (ed.). 2001. *Music, Science, Philosophy: Models in the Universe of Thought*. Aldershot: Ashgate.

Katz, Ruth. 1984. "Collective 'Problem-Solving' in the History of Music: The Case of the Camerata." *Journal of the History of Ideas*, 45: 361–77.

Kemp, Martin. 1990. *The Science of Art: Optical Themes in Western Art from Brunelleschi to Seurat*. New Haven: Yale University Press.

Kenyon, Nicholas (ed.). 1998. *Authenticity and Early Music*. Oxford: Oxford University Press.

Kisby, Fiona (ed.). 2001 "Introduction: Urban History, Musicology and Cities and Towns in Renaissance Europe." In *Music and Musicians in Renaissance Cities and Towns*. Cambridge: Cambridge University Press.

Kramer, Cheryce. 1998. "A Fool's Paradise: The Psychiatry of *Gemüth* in a Biedermeier Asylum." D. Phil. thesis, University of Chicago.

———. 2000a. "Music as a Cause and Cure of Illness in Nineteenth-Century Europe." In Peregrine Horden (ed.), *Music as Medicine: The History of Music Therapy since Antiquity*. Aldershot: Ashgate.

———. 2000b. "Soul Music as Exemplified in Nineteenth-Century German Psychiatry," in P. Gouk (ed.), *Musical Healing*. Aldershot: Ashgate, Aldershot.

Leppert, Richard. 1993. *The Sight of Sound: Music, Representation, and the History of the Body*. Berkeley: University of California Press.

Lindley, Mark. 1984. *Lutes, Viols and Temperaments*. Cambridge: Cambridge University Press.

———. 2001. "Temperaments." In Stanely Sadie (ed.), *The New Grove Dictionary of Music and Musicians*, Vol. 25, 2nd edn. London: Macmillan.

Lindsay, W.M. (ed.). 1911. *Isidori Hispalensis episcopi Etymologiarum sive Originum libri XX*, 2 vols. Oxford: I: K6ʳ

Lowinsky, Edward. 1946. "The Concept of Physical and Musical Space in the Renaissance." *Proceedings of the American Musicological Society*, 57–84.

McClary, Susan. 1998. "Unruly Passions and Courtly Dances: Technologies of the Body in Baroque Music." In Sara E. Melzer and Kathryn Norberg (eds), *From the Royal to the Republican Body: Incorporating the Political in Seventeenth and Eighteenth Century France*. Berkeley: University of California Press.

McGowan, Margaret M. 1963. *L'Art du ballet de cour en France, 1581–1643*. Paris: Editions du Centre National de la Recherche Scientifique.

McLuhan, Marshall. 1962. *The Gutenberg Galaxy*. Toronto: Toronto University Press.

Maurice and Mayer (eds). 1980. *The Clockwork Universe: German Clocks and Automata 1550–1650*. New York: Neale Watson Academic Publishers.

Miller, Leta and Cohen, Albert. 1987. *Music in the Royal Society of London 1660–1806*. Detroit: Information Coordinators.

Moran, Bruce T. 1991a. *The Alchemical World of the German Court: Occult Philosophy and Chemical Medicine in the Circle of Moritz of Hessen (1572–1632)*. Stuttgart: Franz Steiner.

———. (ed.). 1991b. *Patronage and Institutions: Science, Technology and Medicine at the European Court 1500–1750*. Woodbridge: Boydell and Brewer Press.

Moyer, Anne E. 1992. Chapter 1. *Musica Scientia: Musical Scholarship in the Italian Renaissance*. Ithaca and London: Cornell.

New Grove Dictionary of Music. 2001. London: Macmillan.

O'Brien, Grant. 1990. *Ruckers: A Harpsichord and Virginal Building Tradition*. Cambridge: Cambridge University Press.

Ong, Walter. 1958. *Ramus, Method, and the Decay of Dialogue*. Cambridge, MA: Harvard University Press.

Palisca, Claude V. 1960. *Girolamo Mei: Letters on Ancient and Modern Music to Vincenzo Galileo and Giovanni Bardi*. Rome: American Institute of Musicology.

——. 1961. "Scientific Empiricism in Musical Thought." In H. H. Rhys, ed., *Seventeenth-Century Science and the Arts*. Princeton, NJ: Princeton University Press.

——. 1985a. *Humanism in Italian Renaissance Musical Thought*. New Haven: Yale University Press.

——. 1985b "The Science of Sound and Musical Practice." In J.W.Shirley and F.D. Hoeniger (eds), *Science and the Arts*. Washington, London and Toronto: The Folger Shakespeare Library.

Peters, John Durham. 1999. *Speaking into the Air: A History of the Idea of Communication*. Chicago: Chicago University Press.

Poizat, Michel. 1992. *The Angel's Cry: Beyond The Pleasure Principle in Opera*. Trans. Arthur Denner. Ithaca and London: Cornell University Press.

Polk, Keith. 1992. *German Instrumental Music of the Late Middle Ages*. Cambridge: Cambridge University Press.

Porter, Roy (ed.). 1985. *Patients and Practitioners: Lay Perceptions of Medicine in Pre-Industrial Society*. Cambridge: Cambridge University Press.

Rasch, Rudolf. 2002. "Tuning and Temperament." In Thomas Christensen (ed.), *The Cambridge History of Western Music Theory*. Cambridge: Cambridge University Press.

Rastall, Richard. 1983. *The Notation of Western Music: An Introduction*. London: Dent.

Roseman, Marina. 1991. *Healing Sounds of the Malaysian Rainforest: Teimar Music and Medicine*. Berkeley and Los Angeles: University of California Press.

Rousseau, George. 2000. "The Inflected Voice: Attraction and Curative Properties." In P. Gouk (ed.), *Musical Healing in Cultural Contexts*. Ashgate: Aldershot.

Sadie, Stanley (ed.). 1984. *The New Grove Dictionary of Musical Instruments*. 3 vols. London: Macmillan.

Sauveur Joseph. 1984. *Collected Writings on Musical Acoustics*. Ed. Rudolph Rasch. Utrecht: Diapason Press.

Schafer, R. Murray. 1977. *The Soundscape: The Tuning of the World*. Rochester, VT: Destiny Books.

Schmidt, Leigh Eric. 2000. *Hearing Things: Religion, Illusion, and the American Enlightenment*. Cambridge, MA and London: Harvard University Press.

Schullian, Dorothy and Schoen, Max (eds). 1948. *Music and Medicine*. New York: Henry Schuman.

——. 2000. Selected References. In Horden (ed.), *Music as Medicine: The History of Music Therapy since Antiquity*. Aldershot: Ashgate.

Seeger, Anthony. 1987. *Why Suyá Sing: A Musical Anthropology of an Amazonian People*. Cambridge: Cambridge University Press.

Seeger, Anthony. 2002. "Sounds, Social Organization and Cosmology among the Suyá Indians of Mato Grosso, Brazil." Paper presented at the Wenner-Gren International Symposium, Hearing Culture, New Directions in the Anthropology of Sound, April.

Shepherd, John. 1991. *Music as Social Text*. Cambridge: Polity Press and Basil Blackwell.

Shiloah, Amnon (ed.) 1993. *The Dimension of Music in Islamic and Jewish Culture* London: Variorum.

Smith, Bruce R. 1999. "The Soundscapes of Early Modern England." *The Acoustic World of Early Modern England: Attending to the O-Factor*. Chicago: Chicago University Press.

Smith, Mark M. 2004. *Hearing History: A Reader*. Athens, GA: University of Georgia Press.

Stobart, Henry. 2000. "Bodies of Sound and Landscapes of Music: A View from the Bolivian Andes." In P. Gouk (ed.), *Musical Healing in Cultural Contexts*. Aldershot: Ashgate.

Strong, Roy. 1979. *The Renaissance Garden in England*. London: Thames and Hudson.

Tanay, Dorit Esther. 1999. *Noting Music, Marking Culture: The Intellectual Context of Rhythmic Notation, 1250-1400*. Holzgerlingen: Hänssler-Verlag.

Thompson, Emily. 2002. *The Soundscape of Modernity*. Cambridge, MA: MIT Press.

Tinctoris, Johannes. 1975–8. *Opera Theoretica*. 3 vols. Edited by Albert Seay. n.p.: American Institute of Musicology.

Tomlinson, Gary. 1993. *Music in Renaissance Magic: Toward a Historiography of Others*. Chicago: Chicago University Press.

——. 1998. "The Historian, the Performer, and Authentic Meaning in Music." In Nicholas Kenyon (ed.), *Authenticity and Early Music*. Oxford: Oxford University Press.

Truesdell, Clifford A. 1955. "The Theory of Aerial Sound 1687–1788." In *Euleri Opera Omnia*. Lausanne: Birkhauser Verlag.

——. 1960. "The Rational Mechanics of Flexible or Elastic Bodies 1638–1788" In *Euleri Opera Omnia*, 2nd series. Turin.

Van de Wall, Willem. [1948] 2000. "Music in Hospitals." In Dorothy Schullian, and Max Schoen, (eds), *Music and Medicine*. New York: Henry Schuman.

Voss, Angela. 2002. "The Musical Magic of Marsilio Ficino." In Michael J. B. Allen and Valery Rees (eds), *Marsilio Ficino: His Theology, His Philosophy, His Legacy*. Leiden, Boston & Köln: Brill.

Wagner Oettinger, Rebecca. 2001. *Music as Propaganda in the German Reformation*. Aldershot: Ashgate.

Wainwright, Jonathan and Holman, Peter (eds). 2005. *From Renaissance to Baroque: Changes in Instruments and Instrumental Music in the Seventeenth Century*. Aldershot: Ashgate.

Walker, D.P. 1946–7. "The Aims of Baïf's Académie de Poésie et de Musique." *Journal of Renaissance and Baroque Music*, 1: 91–100.

——. 1958. *Spiritual and Demonic Magic from Ficino to Campanella*. London: Warburg Institute.

———. 1972. "Francis Bacon and Spiritus." In Allen G. Debus (ed.), *Science, Medicine and Society in the Renaissance*. New York: Science History Publications. Reprinted with additional notes in Walker, D.P. 1985. *Music, Spirit and Language in the Renaissance*. Ed. Penelope Gouk. London: Variorum.

———. 1978. *Studies in Musical Science in the Late Renaissance*. London: Brill.

———. [1941–2] 1985. "Musical Humanism in the 16th and Early 17th Centuries," *Music, Spirit and Language*. Variorum: London.

Waterhouse, William. 1994. *Dictionary of Musical Wind-Instrument Makers & Inventors*. London: Tony Bingham.

Weber, William. 1992. *The Rise of Musical Classics in Eighteenth-Century England: A Study in Canon, Ritual and Ideology*. Oxford: Clarendon.

Webster, Charles. 1974. *The Great Instauration: Science, Medicine and Reform 1626–1660*. London: Duckworth.

Wegman, Rob C. 1988. "'Das Musikalische Hören,'in the Middle Ages and Renaissance: Perspectives from Pre-War Germany." *Musical Quarterly*, 82 (3/4): 434–54.

West, M. L. 1992. *Ancient Greek Music*. Oxford: Clarendon Press.

Winternitz, Emmanuel. 1979. *Musical Instruments and Their Symbolism in Western Art: Studies in Musical Iconology*, 2nd edn. New Haven: Yale University Press.

———. 1982. *Leonardo Da Vinci as a Musician*. New Haven: Yale University Press.

Woodfield, Ian. 1988. *Early History of the Viol*. Cambridge: Cambridge University Press.

Woolf, Daniel. 1986. "Speech, Text, and Time: The Sense of Hearing and the Sense of the Past in Renaissance England." *Albion*, 18 (2): 159–93.

Yates, Frances. 1947. *French Academies*. London: Warburg Institute.

———. 1969. *The Theatre of the World*. London: Routledge and Kegan Paul.

Fear in Paradise: The Affective Registers of the English Lake District Landscape Re-visited

Divya P. Tolia-Kelly

Divya P. Tolia-Kelly is a cultural geographer at Durham University. She has curated several art exhibitions resulting from research collaborations with visual artists including Graham Lowe and Melanie Carvalho. Her interests include race memory, sensory memory, national heritage, materiality and landscape.
divya.tolia-kelly@durham.ac.uk

ABSTRACT   During the summer of 2004, the artist Graham Lowe and I undertook a research project entitled *Nurturing Ecologies* within the Lake District National Park (LDNP)[1] at Windermere. This landscape, considered as an icon of "Englishness," is revisited through the embodied and sensory experiences of post-migration residents of Lancashire and Cumbria in an attempt to unravel multiple relationships embedded in visitor engagements with this landscape and thus disrupt the moral geography of the landscape as embodying a singular *English* sensibility, normally exclusionary of British multi-ethnic, translocal and mobile landscape values and sensibilities. The research led to the production of a series of drawings and descriptions made in visual workshops by participants, and a set of forty paintings produced by the artist. These paintings are examined in this paper as representing the values, sensory meanings and embodied relationships that exist for migrant communities with this landscape. These groups include the Asian community from the Lancashire town of Burnley and a "mixed" art group living in Lancashire. The initial drawings and subsequent paintings produced operate as a testimony to the Lake District landscape as a site for engendering feelings of terror, fear as well as representing a paradisiacal landscape.

KEYWORDS: sensory landscapes, visual culture, affect, Englishness

Introduction

The English Lake District has been culturally valorized as embodying a space where visitors can engage with a national landscape "sensibility." The "national," in this regard, often slides between being British and English; to simplify matters here, I will refer to these nationally as being England and culturally as inspiring *Englishness*. The participants in the research that formed the basis of this article and their responses to landscape are both situated within England, as residents and through the research process; however, their political citizenship is British. The cultural building blocks of experiencing a national park that orientate the "senses" towards a connection with what it is to be English are made up of visual, aural and literary texts. The Lake District has an identification as a cultural landscape that is iconic through its historical connections with visual artists such as J.M.W. Turner and John Constable, and authors such as Wordsworth and Ruskin. Poetry, painting, art and landscape merge into a textural palimpsest of a recognizable iconographic source of connection with the sensory experiences that these artists responded to and worked through in their art. This "iconography" of Englishness is a "visual space" that also engenders a "structure of feeling" which associates you sensually and artfully to a cultural marker of belonging and being within the historically assembled, national sensibility (Daniels and Cosgrove 1988). I seek, firstly, to engage with the emotional registers of the "structure of feeling" evoked in this landscape in contemporary culture, which make it both an English *place* and simultaneously a textualized "theatre of memory" (Samuel 1989), and, secondly, to investigate the sensory responses that contemporary English visitors have to this palimpsest, including those from communities not typically associated with an Englishness rooted in a national "structure of feeling." Traditionally, these have been figured through a masculinist sensibility (Nash 1996; Rose 1997) and bound up within cultural texts that are collaged to form a singular bounded notion of national culture, formulated as a "moral" landscape of nation (Matless 1998). Green has argued that these landscape values often reflect the "currency of universal and immanent meanings" which occlude historicist analysis and issues of social access and power (1995: 40). The purpose of this article is not to reassert a two-dimensional, singular landscape culture based within the Lake District landscape, but to encourage engagement with this site as a contested landscape the representations and cultural narratives of which are too often figured as excluding multiple histories and affective experiences, including those of gendered and racialized cultural narratives.

The visual methodology used was designed with artist Graham Lowe. Within the visual workshops set up, we sought to explore complex, heterogeneous cultures and sensibilities which also contribute to a modern Englishness that is formed through migrational cultural values from Eastern Europe, the Indian subcontinent, Ireland and Scotland. As Davidson and Bondi (2004) reflect, "whether joyful or heartbreaking, emotion has the power to transfer the shape of our life-worlds ... Creating new fissures and textures we never expected to find." The process of mapping these sensibilities through drawings and paintings traces a set of affective registers that are not normally encountered in representations of this cultural landscape. The visual materials from the research aim to make tangible a divergent set of sensory responses to this landscape and show how affect and emotion are experienced. They show a need for an engagement with the heterogeneity of affectual registers such as "fear" and "terror." The emotional and affectual registers that are represented on canvas are understood as being formed within in specific temporal and spatial fields of experience, beyond singular registers of "fear" and 'terror' (Tolia-Kelly 2006). Firstly, I will outline the relationship between viewing cultural landscapes and emotional connectivity in landscape research. The relationship between vision and emotion, however, is complex, but, by starting with a consideration of the picturesque tradition, I hope to illustrate the value of landscape research which engages with "embodied" and "emotional" cultural engagements in the contemporary English Lake District landscape.

The Picturesque Tradition: Emotion and Landscape Aesthetics

The artist Claude Lorrain has been inspirational to British landscape artists and has said to have inspired J.M.W. Turner's own landscape painting in the early years of his art. Lorrain's work exemplifies the art of the "picturesque." The value and experience of the picturesque landscape can be traced from writers such as Edmond Burke through to William Gilpin, and other painters besides Turner.

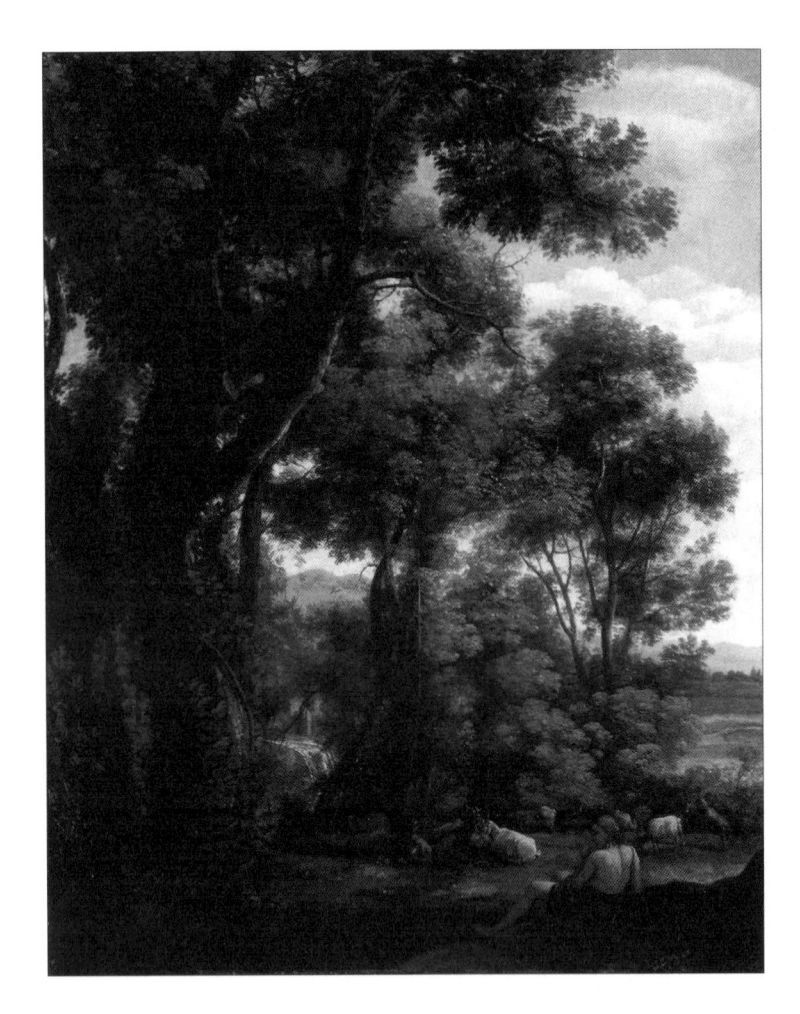

Figure 1
Claude Lorraine (also Géllée) – *Landscape with Goatherds and Goats* (1636). Oil on canvas, 51.4 × 41.3 cm. Courtesy of the National Gallery Picture Library

Picturesque landscape art developed in the eighteenth century between "idealism" in the landscape tradition of the seventeenth century and the Romantic tradition of the nineteenth century. The cultural sensibility of the picturesque tradition is one that celebrated classical cultures, but which simultaneously celebrated nature's wild textures and forms. The roughness and drama of natural forms are framed within a "timeless" perspective. *Landscape with Goatherds* epitomized Claude Lorrain's attitude to nature and form in landscape. The classical forms in this painting set a nostalgic "tone," representing a natural relationship between man, God and nature. Lorraine's paintings reflect the drama of nature through use of scale; often, contrasts between light and dark are reduced to create a sense of distance. Gombrich argues that "it was Claude who first opened people's eyes to the sublime beauty of nature" (1995: 396). In this period, and up to a century after his death, landscape was understood and was "looked for" in the form recognizable through his paintings. As Lorrain's images were encountered in popular culture as sepia replicas, tourists carried with them a black glass lens (Claude Glass) through which to view the scene before them, so that landscape could imitate picture. The engagement with landscape was figured through prior textual encounters. The landscape itself was reshaped to meet the viewer's expectations of form, structure and composition of a site. Nature, in these viewings and experiences was not engaged with in its "natural" rhythms; instead it was carefully choreographed to please the ocular fashions of the day. The relationship between the picturesque viewer and the scene is not figured as an holistic, corporeal engagement, but simply as a process of "picturing." The paintings of Lorrain also inspired Wordsworth in his engagement with the English Lakes; the realism of nature's textures were an inspiration for understanding beauty and led to the Romantic aesthetic in Wordsworth's own art. John Ruskin prized the "wild" qualities reflected in J.M.W. Turner's works, seeing them as representing the "natural fact" of wild nature (Hewison et al. 2000: 28).The distance between the visceral experience and the visual in the picturesque tradition privileges perspective and aesthetics.

Politically, the aesthetics of the picturesque tradition celebrated un-peopled landscapes, or, where there were people, they became part of nature and its rhythms. Darby argues that this tradition valorized the northern landscapes of the Lakes as central to "national" culture situated in the "provincial" spaces of Britain; de-centering the urban cultures of accumulation of wealth and Imperial slavery (2000: 73). The "picturesque" was a precursor to Romanticism, which rejected capitalism, and the encroachment of industry into spaces of the countryside. Aesthetics in Turner's paintings became accentuated representations of earth, sky and sea, without "realism." In Turner's early paintings (for example, see "Barnard Castle" ca.1825) where "nature" is secondary to the forms of architecture of the castle, the aesthetics of the castle are "naturalized" through their depiction through light and a reduction of their form into nodes of light and color. The man-made functionality of the castle is distanced, and the historic stone given life through light. Turner's "northern tour" also challenged the pictorial differences between representations of "south" and "north."

What is occluded in the picturesque tradition is the idea of the dynamism of landscape and emotional values of the cultural landscape. In the picturesque landscape, the sovereignty of the viewer is enabled only through his or her looking with a particular stance, both physically, socially and politically; the relationship between emotional responses to a scene and the form and aesthetics of representation are not of primary value. What is needed is an understanding of aesthetic developments in landscape art that explore the ways in which Turner and others are drawn to this landscape as a result of emotional responses and values. This is linked to positioning the "viewer" as visual commander of the scene (Mitchell 1994; Cosgrove 1984). The picturesque landscape "works" for those with a particular social status: "the center's turn to its own mountainous north, England's Lake District, marks the production of another layer of opposition to that progressive England, as aesthetics and sentiment combined to locate continuity and tradition in the landscape" that denies economic organization of the land and cultural change (Newman 1987: 117, quoted in Darby 2000: 77). As an aesthetic form, the picturesque landscapes of Lorrain and Turner are purely visual. The representations hint at senses of "nostalgia" and "awe" but remain centered on the visual, avoiding reflection upon the corporeal aspect of the encounter, unlike the work of other landscape artists that encourage the viewer to engage with the landscape as a sensual, affective space. England and Englishness is recognizable within this "picturing" of landscape, in which the Lake District landscape became a culturally loaded place, from being empty and desolate (Darby 2000: 54).

The English Lake District has, historically and contemporarily, been the site of the consolidation of an exclusive memorial to a sense of Englishness. This as a site of exclusion, of alienation, and it being a site of multicultural history is a rare narrative. Yet, international flows of people, plants and values of nature present in the landscape shape this cultural space, in the form of place names, for example, and in the grammars and vocabularies of the contemporary tourist economy. The Englishness embedded here is not representative of the history of this site, or the flows of values, memories, narratives and histories that it embodies. It is a landscape made meaningful as site of emotional connectivity. It is a landscape constructed, made meaningful, through multicultural mobility, memory and artifactual registers of engagement – many of these have been held to be "incommunicable" and "intangible," and, as such, impossible to talk about in anything other than abstract terms. These are also those registers that are "not often looked for" in a contemporary or multicultural context. In this research the missing record is readdressed in some small way. The research presented here results from the "Nurturing Ecologies" research project conducted with Graham Lowe which has sought to make tangible these values and embodied relationships with the Lake District landscape. The aim is to give form, through participants' own visual texts and the artist's reflections, to the emotional value of the Lake District landscape to British residents. Before I summarize my research method I want to outline some contemporary tensions concerned with race and exclusion in this iconic landscape.

The Media and Ethnic Englishness in the Lake District

Throughout the summers of 2004 and 2005 several news stories hit the public media that focused on the problem of access to the countryside for ethnic minority communities (Cindi 2004; *Guardian* 2005). There were headlines such as "Country faces 'passive apartheid'" (BBC News Online 2004b) quoting the chairman of the Commission for Racial Equality, Trevor Phillips, who responded to the growing concern over the countryside as being a "white" space. In all of these, the problem was figured as the "nation" being an environment divided along lines of ethnicity, exposing the continuing debates about "rightful belonging" to the English landscape (Parekh 1995; Kinsman 1995). The LDNPA had itself already commissioned several reports in September 2003 to investigate the nature of ethnic minority exclusion and access (Research House UK 2003a; 2003b; 2003c; 2003d). These reports claimed that ethnic minority communities felt disenfranchised from visiting the park and that there were cultural and structural prohibitions to their access and enjoyment of it. These included calls for better and cheaper forms of public transport to the LDNP from local areas and cities. The reports also concluded that many did not have *knowledge* about the park and its facilities. To encourage greater access the LDNPA decided to set aside additional budget for guides for ethnic groups, this was to be done by cutting all tours and guides available for "non-special" visitors. This move by the LDNP caused national controversy, the headlines laid bare a seemingly "cause and effect" decision in favor of encouraging reluctant and uninterested, black and ethnic (and usually urban) visitors at the expense of providing a service for the already enthusiastic, supportive white middle-class visitors. As a result, a private sponsor stepped in to save the threatened services to regular visitors. What this media storm revealed was that arguments that criticized moves to increase attendance by minority ethnic communities were seen to be unnecessary as it was not desirable that these groups be "coerced" into appreciation of this site, also the groups were seen to be a "discordant" market – visually, culturally and socially suspect. Agyeman (1990) argues that the environmental discourses around "non-native belonging" in the English landscape are in tune with cultural discourses that are exclusionary to a black presence in the rural scene. These attitudes reflect the fact that there is "a process of 'containment' is in operation, it keeps black people in certain specified areas" (Agyeman 1990: 233). The research attempted to revisit these ideas and review the claims through group discussions and through recording visitor relationships and values. The Lake District was investigated as being a landscape of nurturing value, and one that held a valued place in the lives of British migrants. Their views, values and responses were recorded within the workshops. Two forms of materials were produced, firstly a set of paintings and visual collages made by the participants of the groups, and, secondly, the set of final paintings produced by Graham Lowe, which are his reflections on the participants work, transcripts and the whole "mapping" process. The paintings are situated within a broader cycle of structures of living as the interpretation of participants' values is achieved through understanding the "positioning" (Hall, 1990) of these groups within British society. Their perceptions and "oppositional" values of "town" and "country" (Williams 1973) are reflected in their materials.

"Doing" Visual Methodologies: Making *Nurturing Ecologies* on Paper

Landscape culture has been rooted within art history, limiting cultures of appreciation to the structures of "aesthetic appreciation" and composition. Engagements with questions of "what do pictures do?" in terms of social and cultural geographies of making art, are limited (Crang 2003). Green has also argued that landscape appreciation has operated within "a strait-jacket which inhibits possibilities for a more effectively historical understanding of landscape" (1995: 33). This is an "elite" cultural lens that excludes everyday, embodied and emotional engagement with landscapes. The design of the methodology used records the appreciation of the visual landscape from a perspective of "everyday folk" and, in particular, the landscape most associated with the visualizing the "national" culture: The English Lake District. The aim was to strive for a set of representations and sensory tracings of the experience of the Lake District for those usually marginal in the national iconography. Working with the landscape artist Graham Lowe afforded the opportunity to record and make tangible some "other" national stories and sensibilities inspired by this landscape. Overall, the research attempts to trace a set of sensory responses to the landscape in a visual mode to enrich the cultural record, and thus extend the variety of "sensibilities" encountered in artistic representations. This process, in the first instance, records migrant sensibilities, and, in the second, through the production of a set of paintings, attempts to redraft the moral geographies of the English Lakes that are usually encountered in the textual cornerstones of Lake District art. The paintings stand as a material contribution to the archives of landscape representations of the varieties of *English* in the story of the cultural values of this iconic landscape. By offering a formal site and space (of the canvas and of the gallery) for the recording of everyday, emotional responses to the Lake District, the production of the final paintings is part of a political process. The canvases, in some small way, add a tangible means both to archive community responses and, more broadly, to contribute to a fuller genealogical picture of the Lake District's "other" histories, and, in particular, its translocal cultural history. The canvases have become part of the art historical economy of Lake District representation, produced by a professional artist.

The texts produced in this research are presented here alongside the contextual process of production – this avoids narrowing "dramatically the field of possibilities through which we might envisage the [cultures of the] visual" beyond representation, but as a force shaping social identity and engagements with nature and landscape itself (Green 1995: 34). The research method aims to ensure that the text becomes the beginning of the process of recording the values of this landscape and not the final product from which art history can delimit meanings and ideas through their simple form.

Thinking and Feeling Landscape through an Inclusive Visual Practice

The artist Graham Lowe and I met in Lancaster in October 2003. Upon discussing landscape art it became clear that we had a mutual interest in memory, everyday values and the material English landscape. We believed that there was a need to investigate other "visions" and examine an alternative perspective and also to record these in canvas form as they were landscape experiences not normally recorded on canvas. This was a new visual practice which would enrich contemporary writing on cultures of landscape which was attentive to embodied, material and affectual registers of landscape values (for example, Wylie 2002; 2005). This mode of engagement often situates the articulator of landscape cultures as sovereign negotiator and empowered explorer of various coherent expressions of landscape as a "performative milieu," or, in Wylie's (2005) terms, negotiations of "a post-phenomenological understanding of the formation and undoing of self and landscape in practice"; he concludes with an idea that "landscape might best be described in terms of the entwined materialities and sensibilities *with which* we act and sense" (p. 245). However, the "we" of these empowered landscape traversings remains a bounded universal body of mobile citizens freed of fear and concerns over racial and/or sexual attack, of the lack of "rightful encounter" with a particular moral geography governing access, and, indeed, free of the chains of childcare, work and the economic constraints to roam. What is necessary in these new theorizations of performative cultures of landscape as practice is an increased acknowledgement of the place of difference and power in shaping the matrices within which "we" can engage with landscape (see also Jazeel 2005). Roaming, in this light, becomes a limited mode of engagement and cannot accommodate landscape cultures for all. In the research design there is a political intention to record multiple cultures of engagement of individuals and groups who are fearful, frail and feel endangered by the concept of even just walking the lakeside pathways of Windermere. Revisiting the sensory values embedded in the landscape with these various modes of engagement in mind incorporates a desire to record emotional values, moving beyond the written text to a multisensorial expression for those who do not have the possibility of accessing this landscape through a visual or literary tradition of English Romanticism with complete sovereignty. The design was aimed to enable a creative process, empowering those who did not write, breaking away from textual expression and with the same stroke breaking the mold of artistic practice and geographical research on landscape to achieve a revisioning of the emotional values of the Lakes and a reimaging of this landscape's sensory registers through, firstly, the representational art of participants in the form of their drawings and collages. These signify sensory values, materially encountered, as they evoke memories of biographical landscapes not normally seen. The aim was also to produce a set of images by a trained artist. In essence, the paintings produced by the artist have captured an alternative emotional citizenry to those sensory registers canonized within this cultural landscape.

The collaboration with the artist was a necessary element of the research design. Initially, the collaboration ensured that there was a professional engagement with the visual, having an artist present as part of the workshop design and the sessions themselves allowed engagement with the notion of producing visual material and valuing the visual. The artist made the process one in which the participants were enabled to produce visual images with attention to form and aesthetics. The presence of an artist shifted the sessions from being about an amateurish research process in which my lack of training would become an obstacle. Moreover, the production of a set of paintings entitled *Nurturing Ecologies/Maps of the Known World* put these individuals' feelings and values in a tangible form in a gallery space. Again, this aim was a political one, intended to place responses in tangible form within the cultural economy of Lake District landscape representations. Some of these canvases have been bought by collections in the towns of Burnley and Lancaster, are now part of local museum displays and have been displayed in the galleries within the National Park itself.

Graham's paintings themselves are, simultaneously, his own reflections and reflections of others' responses: an interpretation of narratives, aesthetic and formal representations in aural, visual and textual modes produced in groups. These are not intended as a process of a "reappropriation" of the participants' views, but one whereby he produced a textual representation on canvas of the relationships with the landscape that were shared with him and had struck a chord in his own artistic psyche. There is a constant circulation of feedback of emotions from and between individuals involved in the process. The result was a collaborative process between participants, Graham and myself in which the participants were involved in exhibitions. Overall, we worked with various participants – around eighty in all, at Windermere over a period of six weeks in the summer of 2004. To enable a trusting group dynamic we recruited "ready made" groups of people living in Lancashire and Cumbria. The first was from the *Pakistan Welfare Association* (based in Burnley), which welcomed opportunities for "activities" and "trips" and was keen to be involved in something beyond research about "the negatives" of race riots in Burnley in 2000–1. The recruitment meetings attracted around forty participants; we recruited two groups of twenty-two men (in age all were in their forties and fifties) and twenty-two women (all aged in their late thirties up to their mid-fifties). We appointed a male and a female translator to suit the requirements of the single sex groups. We then recruited an "art group" that Graham had led at a community college. The art group was a mixed group of around five men (aged from twenty-one to forty) and twelve women (aged from thirty-eight to sixty).

Our first workshop was held at Littledale Hall. Here, we had a taste of the Lake District environment. There was a dining room and a large lounge space to accommodate thirty people; the space provided the opportunity to enhance the scope for "liminality" (see Burgess et al. 1988a and 1988b). At Littledale we held two activities. We first asked the group about their biographical relationships with past landscapes and present ones. A "collective" biography came through: in the Burnley group, the men and women had similar routes to each other, although they had not traveled together; the environments in which they now lived and those left behind in Pakistan were the same, however. The Burnley group had migrated from Gujarat in Pakistan, named after the Indian state from which their families had been during Partition. Gujarat in Pakistan lies on the foothills of the Himalayas; it is a rural district made up of scores of hamlets where subsidence farming is in practice. Graham's "art group" similarly had a group identity, based around their relationship with art. In the biography sessions, men of the group talked through their "values" of the Lakes and many complained that it was difficult to escape "armchair" tourism and access *real* landscapes or nature.

In the afternoon, visual workshop we asked the groups to produce a visual collage of their valued landscapes. Using pictures in books, magazines such as the *National Geographic* that contained several types of landscapes from all over the world including from Pakistan, India, Eastern Europe, Britain and African nations, the group created familiar landscapes. A week later the groups met again and traveled to Windermere. We took the groups on a short walk to Rydal Water, and had a discussion session over coffee at the Brockhole Visitors Centre overlooking Lake Windermere; then, in the afternoon, we had lunch at St Martin's College in Ambleside. We had facilities for all – a prayer room, refreshments, washing facilities and a room with a panoramic window overlooking Windermere. In these sessions we asked the groups to record (using paint and paper) their responses to their experience of the Lake District. The aim was to discover their responses to the landscape to gain insight into how this landscape *feels* to the groups.

Why a Visual Method? What do the Paintings Offer?

The design of our methodology was aimed to enhance the possibilities for *multivocality*. Halliday argues that innovative visual methodologies can counter the traditional power dynamics of other methods, but require continued reflection on whether their aim is to "further legitimate the *truth* of the research itself." (2000: 504). Pink (2001), in response, argues for reflexive modes of representing participant "voices." Here, the images are *situated* within a biographical context (both in my own papers and in the gallery space in the form of a poster), and the process of production is outlined as transparently as is possible. The images represent the way people experience the Lake District landscape and the assumption here is that seeing is embodied, figured through the cultural lens through which we experience environment. We cannot "see" and "feel" separately; my argument here is that aesthetics in representations are about emotions as much as they are about form, visual grammars permeate with visceral narrations of embodied values. In the picturesque tradition, as a "see-er" you were commanding the landscape; however, everyday landscape experience does not embody such a powerful positioning. This is where "embodied" seeing can be the only way to make sense of cultures of experiencing landscape. We do not simply feel as *context* to seeing, but see through an embodied, feeling engagement. This is why these images are about "feeling" as much as they are about representation, narration or the geopolitics of being English and *other* in a space of narrating the national cultural sensibility. Kearnes supports this further: "One does not simply see ... objects and phenomena are *seeable* or *visible* ... in machinic combination with discourses, knowledges and spaces" (2000: 335). The paintings, when exhibited, do function as representations, but as a revisioning of a national iconography through multiple sensory encounters not normally visualized on canvas. It has been important to design the visual workshops to maximize participation, not to delimit responses through the use of formal English. Visual methods that are designed to include discussions in multiple languages offer a means of "triangulation" of methods; in the case of the Burnley group this allowed the space to be *owned* by those speaking Urdu, Punjabi or Hindi. This move towards working in a multilingual space beyond "English" opened up the possibility for forging more even relationships within the group and making the "doing" of art and painting possible. The use of art materials served to contribute to forcing the groups to work beyond their normal formal grammars and communications about landscape. The paints and paper allowed us to attempt to set up activities which were about capturing alternative vocabularies and visual grammars that are not always encountered or expressible in oral interviews. In previous research it has been difficult to persuade usually more conservative South Asian groups to talk about abstract environmental values. The process of abstracting "environmental values," "emotional values" and "aesthetic responses" was assisted by being at Windermere and through the visual and physical practice – including the unusual physical actions of using hands, fingers and arms differently than in the day-to-day (Bingley 2003).

Although there are disadvantages to using my particular visual methodology in the ways that I have outlined, there are, equally, problems with other visual methods. Other methodologies, such as photography and auto-ethnographic approaches to embodied landscape practice, do offer alternative routes, but for me the critical notion of "positioning" is better explored in the group process, and the production of an exhibition of works at the end of the research was also critical. In practical terms, problems included getting people relaxed enough to paint – this can be a psychological mine field. We avoided problems in this regard in the recruitment of ready-made art-groups or those enthusiastic about the method itself, also we planned to ensure that we maximized "liminality" in the workshop spaces. Even after these precautions were taken, the methodology was still tricky, as encouraging people to paint or draw or talk about landscape and emotions inevitably is. The Burnley men were particularly resistant; some felt embarrassed and regarded "doing art" as "feminine" and did not represent "modernity." Thus, some men were wary of being associated with something "rustic." Graham took photographs and assisted, some directed him to mix colors, others to draw and paint objects with which they had struggled. The sessions were tape-recorded and together these visual and aural texts formed the basis to Graham's paintings. Forty were produced over eighteen months from September 2004 to April 2006. Within this period there were four gallery exhibitions held at the Duke's Theatre Gallery (2004), Townley Hall Museum Gallery in Burnley, the "Fear" conference at the University of Durham (2005), and the Theatre by the Lake (2006), Keswick. In the next section I want to analyze the meanings embedded in these paintings.

Representing Emotional Geographies of the Park: Interpretations on Canvas

The three images in Figures 2–4 are examples of a counter-landscape aesthetic formed by Graham Lowe in his interpretations of the group's responses. In this section I have reflected Graham's explanation of the production of this set of images. The paintings produced were created using a soft pastel and liquid acrylic. His aim was to produce small intimate images (32 cm^2) which would help to express the emotions being discussed in the group sessions. He was aiming to express something of the response of the participants in the groups to the landscape. In Graham's view, the canvas itself "creates a site for the imagination," a place in which, perhaps, the viewer's emotions may be garnered and indeed mirrored. At the exhibition in Lancaster, some of the viewers discussed fear and anxiety when viewing the paintings' "isolation" and "remembered landscape." They resonated with them through the form and palette. Graham worked with material in different forms, (visual, textual and aural); this was overwhelming at first, but helpful in getting a depth of understanding of the landscape values recorded in the sessions.

Isolation is based on Boris. In the workshop he compared the LDNP to the area in which he lives: the outskirts of a small village, a landscape of isolation and anxiety. A landscape in which there is

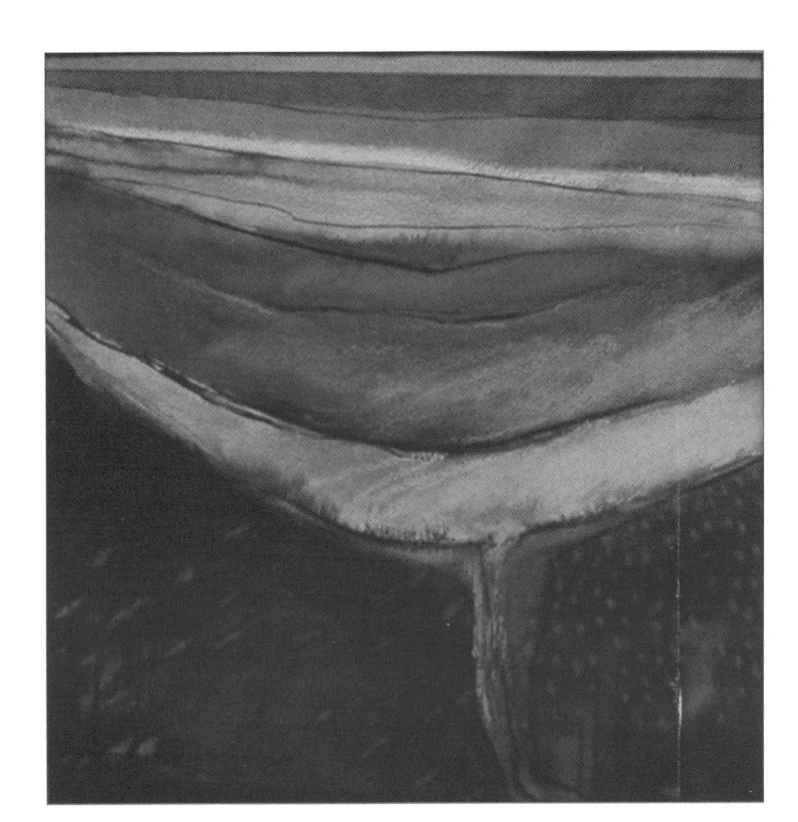

Figure 2
Graham Lowe – *Isolation* (2005)

space to reflect. He says "You can't get away from yourself, you are faced with yourself, and there is a lack of diversions. If you are emotionally or psychologically in a bad place all sorts of fears and anxieties come up." In an interview about the painting, Graham states that in it "I have tried to capture the essence of his statement." To this end, within the painting there are no trees, no landmarks and no points of reference. Boris talked of his fears and anxieties which, as he put it, *came up* during his visit to Windermere. The marks at the bottom reflect the *rising up* of these anxieties- "rising up like bubbles in a glass." Boris's fear is caused by being in the landscape, this is a catalyst to his facing his own anxieties, and he cannot escape these when he is in this space. Boris, in this encounter, is not engaged with a "national" landscape, his experience is counter to that of Lorrain's followers and different to usual responses to Turner's popular scenes. His claustrophobia is encountered as an individual emotion in the landscape of the Lakes. He is sensitized and fearful when the landscape is bare, un-peopled and non-utilitarian.

In his painting *Safe in Dark Places* Graham reflects on Sam's comments on how he felt safer in the dark places of the lakes, in the forests. He loves tree roots, the rocks and mosses "the grubby, spotty spaces." Sam feels fear of the open spaces, when in the

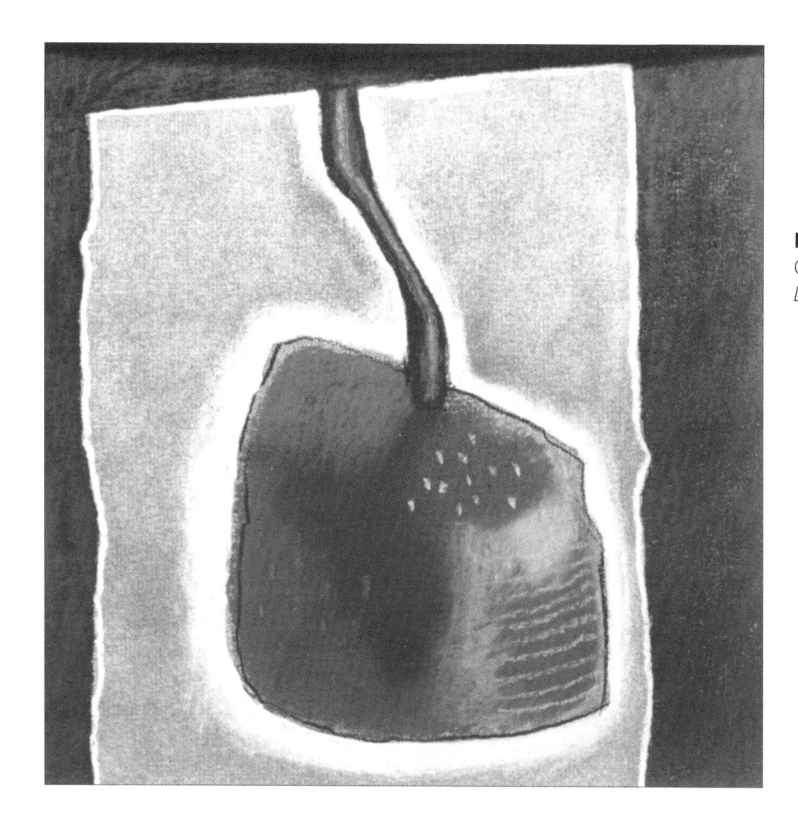

Figure 3
Graham Lowe – *Safe in Dark Places* (2005)

open he feels unanchored, vulnerable to attack. In the painting, the light area is surrounded on three sides by a dark border. The object in the center, literally the grubby spotty, space, appears to be three dimensional, a container. This is like a womb-like space with a life-line, an umbilical cord that links him to the outside world like a tree root. This is, for Sam, the place in which to feel safe. This painting is made reflecting Sam's own picture, which is a dark, black mass of paint with little color and few lines. On seeing this image the group responded with shock and surprise at his response to the paradisiacal beauty of the surrounding landscape. Sam craved the safety of enclosure, the safety of organic matter away from an objective perspective over vistas and panoramas of the Lakeland fells. The scale of the landscape to which he retreats reflects his feelings of safety in the usually unseen textures of soil, branches, bark and moss at the ground level of landscape encounter – the soil that is not often seen, or looked for, in trips to the Lakes is a picture of safety.

In *Fear of High Places* Graham has reflected on the discussion he had with the Burnley women at Windermere. Many expressed their delight at the surroundings; describing it as a landscape of *paradise*. In response to this, Graham suggested taking them to the

Divya P. Tolia-Kelly

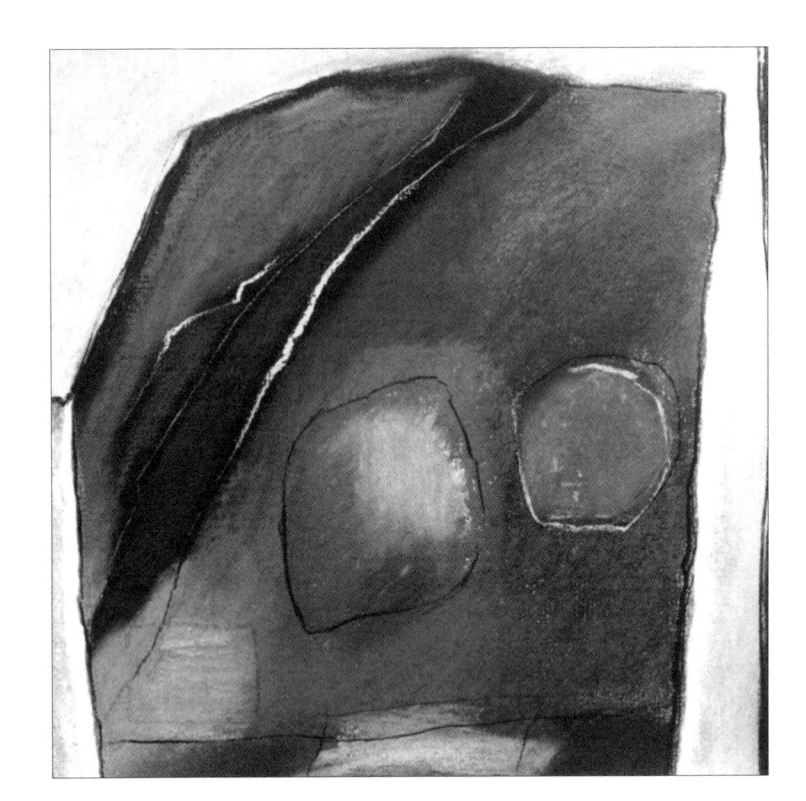

Figure 4
Graham Lowe – *Fear of High Places* (2005)

top of Kirkstone Pass with a steep view of the valley. The women's group became visibly anxious and, without exception, refused to go. They experienced collective anxiety. The interpreter stated that they were "afraid to venture into a high wilderness landscape." Their anxiety was evident from their body language and the tone of their conversations. In Graham's painting he interprets this fear as a barrier blocking their access into these high places. The women fear the very type of landscape walking that Wylie (2005) embarks upon. The physical act of walking the open pathways is a frightful prospect and reflects a counter to the (usually) masculinist (Nash 1996) impulses to conquer views from the highest viewing point. The women were comfortable at low ground, in a group and in a *social* group experience of this landscape. Yasmin describes being completely overwhelmed by the mountains "I felt very small, isolated and fearful in these surroundings." In this painting Graham has tried to express these feelings in the use of composition and color:

> The mainly dark shape dominates the picture plain, with a dark and brooding sky above. The only relief from the somber colors is the yellow area to the right which reflects my observations of the ever changing light in mountain landscape.

Here, the "awe" inspired by this picturesque landscape is experienced as terror in Yasmin's account; the very act of viewing and picturing the scene engenders fright. This is, again, counter to the eighteenth-century practice of *seeing* beauty and awe in the majesty of these mountains.

Initially, Graham found creating this body of work to be extremely challenging. Creating paintings which originated in discussions was novel. Also, working with others, whose experience of landscape was often very different than his own, was stimulating but also stirred up emotions that he himself was not expecting; working with émigrés and poverty stricken migrants from rural Pakistan was heart wrenching. It took a while for Graham to settle with a style, to find a way of producing successful images that would engage with the viewer and create a dialogue which expressed something of the emotions that were discussed in the groups. As a set of images they represent landscapes that are far from the "picturesque" mode of Lorrain's art. They show as everyday emotions such as "fear," "awe," "terror" and "pain." The paintings encompass a visual grammar of landscape produced by the groups. Graham's training in abstract art, and his use of lines and block color, renders them intimate, immediate and accessible. The audience is invited to reflect on the emotional landscape and respond to the embedded registers of fear.

Locating the Fear of Paradise

There is a relationship between emotional registers and landscape culture that shapes the politics of identity and cultures of landscape simultaneously. In understanding the moral geographies of landscapes such as the English Lake District we need not simply attend to the matter of "adding emotions" to existing accounts. Instead, my aim is to show how the feelings that mobility affords – freedom, connection and disconnection, new opportunities for self-expression, loneliness and family stress – are implicated in the experiential texture of transnational experiences. My premise here is that the emotional dimensions of transnational mobility shape experiences of place. Tracing these may bring us some way towards understanding, recording and critically reflecting on the cultures of landscape and mobile citizenship that is not "local." This is an issue of increasing importance in an age of increasing migration, displacement and mobility for those not deemed "local." As Mitchell (2001) has argued, embedded in cultures of national identity is a "lure of the local." It "is not a lure of myths through which people make sense of their own lives, but the lure of mythologies through which power is consolidated and solidified, and the project of racism is advanced" (p. 277).

The Burnley group's perceptions of the Lake District landscape, reveal a "relational" valuing of this fecund "paradise" against the oppressive, ecologically barren and economically denuded Burnley city landscape. Through including these experiences as part of my interpretation, I aim to enrich the research process and, in turn, provide a "whole" picture, rather than reducing the minority ethnic experience as always relating to their urban social life. The communities' valuing of the landscape of Gujarat in Pakistan, are also embedded in their responses to the LDNP through memory. The Burnley women's fear resonated with their lack of "know-how" in this environment: they felt disorientated by the new landscape, unknown to them. Experiences of fear were present in their own "community" space, yet a desire for enfranchisement was less in a space that represented for them a "fear of high places." Their sentiments troubled me, as this group had lived in the Himalayan foothills, their "high places" were one hundred fold higher and steeper. The Burnley group within the landscape of the Himalayas, in contrast to the Lakes, were not carrying a portmanteau of lost dreams and lives; their lives here are complex, as "we stay for our children" is a common claim. Some of the women's paintings show lush kitchen-gardens in Pakistan, where they lived in a cultivated landscape. They describe the ease of moving through this landscape, whereas in the UK they are shut in – as the space around is not solely for their kith and kin they risk being suspected of dishonor more easily if seen without their spouse. Since many of the women have lost their husbands to respiratory illnesses and heart disease (as a result of poor working conditions in the mill factories), they have little choice but to stay at home with children. Their fear in the Lakes reflected physical insecurities in unfamiliar surroundings; a lack of Halal food, prayer rooms, water, distance familiarity and racism were all stated as contributing to their fears. Their incongruity was also a source of anxiety, however, this is not limited to Windermere but extends to the towns of Nelson and Burnley too. Racism was constantly referred to in the group conversations. On reading the Burnley landscape it was easy to see that the women had been isolated further since the riots, their alienation and oppression had increased. Many of their drawings show dark rooms, with windows looking out. These women felt despondent about their children's future. The Burnley men, too, found it difficult to talk about their past rural village life, and were even more silent on their present lives. At home they had difficulty filling their days; with limited possibilities of work they attended the community center to read newspapers and attend the luncheon club. In Burnley, the Asians certainly experience racist violence and fear for the future welfare of their community. Ahmed (2004a; 2004b) argues for the imperatives of racial violence to be understood as emotionally driven, her argument focuses on the collectivity of emotional imperatives for both sides of the race line:

> We can consider racism as a particular form of inter-corporeal encounter: a white racist subject who encounters a racial other may experience an intensity of emotions (fear, hate, disgust,

pain). That intensification involves moving away from the body of the other, or moving towards that body in an act of violence.
(Ahmed 2004b)

For the Burnley community, corporeal engagements with landscape are constantly figured through racialized, geopolitical positionings; the fears expressed here reflect their pormanteau of the way their landscape experiences are transposed elsewhere. However, their registers of fear are just one element of the fears that the Lake District landscape evokes in the participants. Differential registers for "fear" are critical here; Sam's experience of fear, although resonating with collective social fears about attack and vulnerability, is not about a transpersonal, affective experience. Sam feared open spaces because he felt a physical vulnerability to violence as an individual: he is terrified of personal attack. For him, the awesome landscape did not present a fear of a "sublime" landscape; his sublime was in the details of close inspection of woodland, tracing patterns in the mosses, bark and humus. Sam describes his joy on encountering microscale landscape: "Well incidental, they're incidental joys I always think because they're there just doing their thing ... I do, do dark things ... I zoomed in on sort of square foot underneath the bottom of a tree."

Sam's incidental joy, inspired by the comment "you have brought me to heaven," made by some of the Muslim women at Brockhole, is operating on very different registers of exhilaration, thus, the scale of joy, the location of the experience and understandings alone are not sufficient to think through the value of "joyous" spaces in this landscape. I would argue that there is a need to retheorize affectual registers through understanding the situation of the body that experiences these emotions. Emotional registers shape landscape and geographies of identification. By considering the social experiences of empowerment, occlusion, marginality, transnationalism and alienation we can develop a nuanced approach to varied affectual geographies, treating registers of affect as multilayered occurrences of "fear" and "joy." Sensitivity towards vernacular landscapes and power geometries can only enrich current landscape research.

Conclusion
This paper is a reflection on the expression of fear, terror, and anxiety garnered in the *Nurturing Ecologies* research project and the resulting representations on the canvases produced by the artist Graham Lowe. These make tangible the alternative sensibilities that this landscape engenders in varied "English" folk visiting this space: "other" British folk, with a right to peaceful enjoyment. It has been really important to record various responses to the English Lake District, despite my reservations about situating "cultures" as bounded, geographical and social frames these do serve as a starting point for genealogical research that uncovers lost or hidden voices. The canvases are a

set of the visualizations of landscape cultures in the Lake District that have been a response to historical and canonized narrations. In this regard, I have also sought to trouble the affectual approach to social science research by insisting that "race" and power figure in the possibilities of affectual encounter, but also form social identities and, in turn, social landscapes (Hemmings 2005). The Burnley group experience the LDNP as a "sublime" landscape that reflects God's work on Earth, their feelings cultivated through religious values rooted in the Q'ran. The landscape of the Lakes remains a place of sensory engagement – joyful and fearful; however, understanding these affective registers as figured through socially contextual power geometries enhances the value of geographies of emotion and affect. Understanding emotions in different registers linked to "structures of feeling" shaped by a national moral politics allows us to increase understandings of twenty-first-century English sensibilities, including those experienced by the "mobile" English, migrants and communities of visitors that form the maelstrom of material practices that carve out the modern Lake District experience. Wordsworth, in his own guide to the Lake District, describes it as being "a sort of national property, in which every man has a right and an interest who has an eye to perceive and a heart to enjoy" (quoted in Matless 1998: 251). This right continues to be struggled over, not simply in terms of access, but in terms of what possibilities of engagement a national culture of landscape could allow. If "national culture" was to be determined through a broader lens of what constitutes "national landscape," Wordsworth's humanistic utopianism could be afforded to all of today's visitors who experience various registers of terror, fear, and joy.

This research is within the realms of cultural and moral geographies of the English landscape, aimed at advancing the research being conducted on environmental values held by migratory groups in Britain.

Acknowledgment

The *Nurturing Ecologies* project was generously funded by Lancaster University in the summer of 2004.

Note

1. The Lake District National Park is the official name of the National Park within which Windermere is situated. It is managed by the Lake District National Park Authority.

References

Agyeman, J. 1990. "Black People in a White Landscape: Social and Environmental Justice." *Built Environment*, 16:232–6.

Ahmed, S. 2004a. "Collective Feelings: or the Impressions Left by Others." *Theory, Culture And Society*, 21:25–42.

———. 2004b. "Affective Economies." *Social Text*, 22(2): 117–39.

Anderson, K. and Smith, S.J. 2001. "Emotional Geographies." *Transactions of the Institute of British Geographers*. 26: 7–10.

Bingley, A.D. 2003. "In Here and Out There: Sensations between Self and Landscape." *Social and Cultural Geography*, 4(3): 329–45.

BBC News UK, 2004, "Country Faces 'Passive Apartheid." *BBC News Online*, October 8, 2003. http://News.Bbc.Co.Uk/1/Hi/Uk/3725524.Stm (accessed October, 2004).

Burgess, J., Limb, M. and Harrison, C. 1988a "Exploring Environmental Values through the Medium of Small Groups: 1. Theory and Practice." *Environment and Planning*, 20: 309–26.

——. 1988b "Exploring Environmental Values through the Medium of Small Groups: 2. Illustrations of a Group at Work." *Environment and Planning A* 20: 457–76.

Cosgrove, D. 1984. *Social Formation and Symbolic Landscape*. London: Croom Helm.

Cosgrove, D. and Daniels, S. 1988. *The Iconography of Landscape*. Cambridge: Cambridge University Press.

Crang, M. 2003. "Qualitative Methods: Touchy, Feely, Look-See?" *Progress in Human Geography*, 27:494–504.

Darby, W. J. 2000. *Landscape and Identity: Geographies of Nation and Class*. London: Berg.

Davidson, J. and Bondi, L. 2004. "Spatialising Affect; Affecting Space: An Introduction." *Gender, Place and Culture*, 11: 373–4.

Gilroy, P. 1987. *There Ain't No Black in the Union Jack*. London: Routledge.

Gombrich, E. 1995 [first published 1950]. *The Story of Art* London: Phaidon.

Green, N. 1995. "Looking at the Landscape." In Eric Hirsch And Michael

O'Hanlon (eds), *The Anthropology of Landscape*. Oxford: Oxford University Press.

Guardian, The. 2005. "National Parks are the Domain of the White Middle Class." January 12.

Hall, S. 1990. "Cultural Identity and Diaspora." In John Rutherford (ed.), *Identity: Community Culture and Difference*. London: Lawrence and Wishart.

Halliday, R. 2000. "We've Been Framed: Visual Methodology." *The Sociological Review,* 48: 503–21.

Hemmings, C. 2005. "Invoking Affect: Cultural Theory and the Ontological Turn." *Cultural Studies*, 19: 548–67.

Hewison, R. Worrell, I. and Wildman, S. 2000. *Ruskin, Turner and The Pre-Raphaelites* London: Tate Gallery Publishing.

Jazeel, T. 2005. "'Nature', Nationhood and the Poetics of Meaning in Rahuna (Yala) National Park, Sri Lanka." *Cultural Geographies*, 12:199–227.

John, Cindi. 2003. "Black Projects Target Green Pastures." *BBC News UK*, October 8, 2003, http://News.Bbc.Co.Uk/1/Hi/Uk/3590658.Stm (accessed October, 2004).

Kearnes, M. 2000. "Seeing is Believing is Knowing: Towards a Critique of Pure Vision." *Australian Geographical Studies*, 38: 332–40.

Kinsman, P. 1995. "Landscape, Race and National Identity: The Photography of Ingrid Pollard." *Area*, 27: 300–10.

Matless, D. 1995. "The Art of Right Living." In Steve Pile And Nigel Thrift (eds), *Mapping The Subject*. London: Routledge, pp. 93–122.

———. 1997. "Moral Geographies of English Landscape." *Landscape Research*, 22:141–55.

———. 1998. *Landscape and Englishness*. London: Reaktion.

Nash, C. 1996. "Reclaiming Vision: Looking at Landscape and the Body." *Gender, Place and Culture*, 3: 149–69.

Mitchell, W.J.T. 1994. *Landscape and Power*. Chicago: Chicago University Press.

———. 2001. "The Lure of the Local: Landscape Studies at the End of a Troubled Century." *Progress in Human* Geography, 25: 269–81.

Mitchell, W.J.T. 1989. *Landscape and Power*. Chicago and London: University of Chicago Press.

Parekh, B. 1995. "The Concept of National Identity." *New Community*, 21: 255–68.

Pink, S. 2001. "More Visualising, More Methodologies: On Video, Reflexivity and Qualitative Research." *The Sociological Review*, 49, 586–99.

Research House UK. 2003a. *The Mosaic Project: Focus Groups held with the Bangladeshi and Iranian Community from Newcastle who Visited the LDNP*. Report commissioned by the Lake District National Park Authority and the Countryside Agency.

———. 2003b. *The Mosaic Project: Focus Groups held with El-Siddai Outreach Ministries Pre and Post Visit to the LDNP*. Report commissioned by the Lake District National Park Authority and the Countryside Agency.

———. 2003c. *The Mosaic Project: Focus Groups held with Nguzo Saba Group from Preston who Visited LDNP*. Report commissioned by the Lake District National Park Authority and the Countryside Agency.

———. 2003d. *The Mosaic Project: Focus Groups held with the Wai Yin Group from Manchester who Visited the LDNP*. Report commissioned by the Lake District National Park Authority and the Countryside Agency.

Rose, G. 1997. "Feminist Geographies of Environment, Nature and Landscape." In G. Rose, V. Kennard, M. Morris and C. Nash (eds), *Feminist Geographies*. London: Longman.

Samuel, R. 1989. *Theatres of Memory*. London: Verso.

Schama, S. 1996. *Landscape and Memory*. Pennsylvannia: Harper Perrenial.

Tolia-Kelly, D.P. 2006. "Affect – An Ethnocentric Encounter?: Exploring the 'Universalist' Imperative of Emotional/Affectual Geographies." *Area*, 38 (2): 213–7.

Williams, R. 1973. *The Country and the City*. London: Hogarth Press.

Wylie, J. 2002. "An Essay in Ascending Glastonbury Tor." *Geoforum*, 33 (4): 441–54.

———. 2005. "A Single Day's Walking: Narrating Self and Landscape on the South West Coast Path." *Transactions of the Institute of British Geographers*, 30: 234–47.

call for papers

PHOTOGRAPHY & CULTURE

NEW JOURNAL IN 2008

Photography & Culture is a new refereed journal that will be international in its scope and inter-disciplinary in its contributions. It aims to interrogate the contextual and historic breadth of photographic practice from a range of informed perspectives and to encourage new insights into the media through original and incisive writing.

Photography & Culture will publish research papers, discursive critiques and reviews. It will appear at a key moment as photography evolves; once again, to embrace a technological change that is shifting both contemporary usage and historic understanding.

Photography & Culture will quickly establish itself as the leading platform for critical thinking on photography and as essential reading the world over for academics, curators and practitioners with a central and indeed tangential interest in the media.

Editors

Val Williams
University of the Arts, Photography and the Archive Research Centre at London College of Communication, UK

Kathy Kubicki
University College for the Creative Arts at Farnham, UK

Alison Nordström
George Eastman House, USA

Photography & Culture is now seeking articles for early issues of the journal and the editors invite the following submissions:

- **Articles** (3000-5000 words)
- **Discursive Critiques and Research Papers** (1500-4000 words)
- **Reviews** (800-1500 words)

Please email your idea or proposal to the address below for advice before submitting completed pieces. Submissions will be reviewed anonymously by at least two referees. The journal will use the Harvard referencing system with author's name and date incorporated into the text and a full reference in alphabetical order at the end of the article.

All submissions should be sent electronically as Microsoft Word documents to:

submitjournal@photographyresearchcentre.co.uk

BERG

Surprising the Senses

Geke D.S. Ludden, Hendrik N.J. Schifferstein and Paul Hekkert

Geke D.S. Ludden is a Ph.D. candidate at the Department of Industrial Design of Delft University of Technology. Her research focuses on how sensory perception influences the experience of products.
g.d.s.ludden@tudelft.nl

Hendrik N.J. Schifferstein is Associate Professor at the Department of Industrial Design of Delft University of Technology studying the multisensory experiences evoked by consumer durables.
h.n.j.schifferstein@tudelft.nl

Paul Hekkert is Professor of Form Theory at the faculty of Industrial Design Engineering, Delft University of Technology and head of the section Design Aesthetics.
p.p.m.hekkert@tudelft.nl

ABSTRACT We perceive the world around us and the objects in it with all our senses. Designers can therefore influence the way we experience everyday products by paying attention to the multiple sensory aspects of products.

When sensory information from two or more senses conflicts, people can be surprised. Currently, more and more product designers are experimenting with designing products that provide incongruent sensory information. Creating such products enables these designers to evoke interest for their products and let people experience something new.

In several studies, we have investigated people's reactions to and opinions about products with sensory incongruities. The results of our studies suggest that evoking surprise by incorporating sensory incongruities in products can be seen as a means to create more pleasurable product experiences.

KEYWORDS: senses, incongruity, product design

People use products at virtually every moment of the day – and, while doing so, they continually experience these products through multiple senses. For example, when I put on my wristwatch in the morning I see the simple and straight lines it has, I can smell the leather of the strap, I feel the cold steel of the casing on my skin and if I put the watch against my ear I can hear the clockwork ticking. All these perceptions provide me with information about my watch and can influence how I experience my watch. The sound tells me if my watch is still functioning, the pleasant leather smell brings back memories and I enjoy looking at the simple shape.

The preceding example illustrates that product designers can influence the way people experience products by paying attention to the multiple sensory aspects of product design: when visual, tactual, auditory and olfactory aspects all contribute to the experience, together they create a rich form of user–product interaction (MacDonald 2001; Rashid 2003). New and smart(er) materials offer wide opportunities for designers to explore new sensory experiences (Verbücken 2003: 54–9). Many designers recognize the possibilities of new materials and apply them to their designs. In some cases designers make a product that provides incongruent information to different senses. Someone who perceives a product does not necessarily receive all sensory information at the same time. Therefore, perceiving one sensory aspect of a product first can create an expectation of what will be perceived through other sense modalities. The information perceived consecutively may disconfirm the expectation formed upon the initial perception, resulting in a surprise reaction.

Designers can deliberately try to evoke a surprise reaction, because it captures attention to the product, leading to increased product recollection and recognition, and to increased word-of-mouth advertising (Derbaix and Vanhamme 2003; Lindgreen and Vanhamme 2003). The product user may also benefit from sensory incongruity in a product, because it makes the product potentially more interesting to interact with. In addition, experiencing incongruity often involves learning something new about a product or about a particular aspect of a product, such as the material it is made of.

Some forms of sensory incongruity are more likely to occur than others. The senses can be divided into two groups: the distance senses, which are audition, vision and olfaction and the proximity senses, which are taste and touch. People are capable of seeing, hearing and smelling objects from a distance, but in order to touch or taste something, people have to be in physical contact with the object. Therefore, it is more likely that a person will perceive an object through vision, audition, or olfaction first. Furthermore, among the three distance senses, vision provides the most detailed information about a product within the shortest time frame (Jones and O'Neil 1985; Schifferstein and Cleiren 2005). Therefore, sensory incongruities that start with a visual impression are most likely to occur under natural circumstances and, therefore, seem the most relevant for product design.

In several studies (Ludden and Schifferstein n.d., n.d.[2]; Ludden et al. n.d.), we have inspected people's reactions to and opinions about visual–tactual, visual–auditory and visual–olfactory incongruities in products. Among these, visual–tactual incongruities are a special case because the same product attributes can be perceived through both these senses: people can both see and feel a shape or a texture. Visual–auditory and visual–olfactory incongruities always involve multiple product attributes: people cannot see an odor or a sound. However, when someone sees a small product, he or she may expect it to make a high-pitched sound, and when someone sees a pink object, he or she may expect it to have a sweet smell. Therefore, experiencing visual–olfactory and visual–auditory incongruities probably occurs through cognitive association rather than through direct perception.

When we asked consumers in focus groups to talk about examples of sensory incongruity from their own experience, visual–tactual incongruities were mentioned most often (Ludden et al. 2006). For example, several participants mentioned benches that were softer than expected:

> I was at a museum once, where I saw a bench that looked like a rock. I really thought I would be sitting down on a rock but when I did, the rock appeared to be soft. I thought this was funny.

Most of the surprises experienced through sensory incongruity were evaluated positively (funny, comfortable, pleasant). Participants mentioned that they liked experiencing sensory incongruity at times when they were bored (for example, in waiting rooms and public spaces). Some participants mentioned that they would not want to own products with sensory incongruities because they expected the surprise to become boring in the long-term: "I think all these things will become boring with time, even if they are fun at first, after a couple of times it becomes irritating, so it's not fun to have them." However, others mentioned that they would like to own such products to be able to show them to other people: "I think it is fun to have this (surprisingly soft bench) in your home because every time someone new comes in and sits on it they experience the same."

The difference between visual–tactual incongruity on the one hand and visual–olfactory and visual–auditory incongruity on the other hand seems to have consequences for how people experience these incongruities. Our studies suggest that people are more often surprised by visual–tactual incongruities. At the same time, an analysis of contemporary product designs presented in five issues of *The International Design Yearbook* (de Lucchi and Hudson 2001; Lovegrove and Hudson 2002; Maurer and Andrew 2000; Morrison et al. 1999; Rashid 2003) showed that using this form of sensory incongruity in products is not uncommon. Knowingly or not, considerable numbers of designers create visual–tactual incongruities in products, and, while doing so, they seem to use different design strategies (Ludden et al. 2007).

On the basis of an analysis of 101 products exhibiting visual–tactual incongruities, we distinguished two types of surprising products, "Hidden Novelty" (HN) and "Visible Novelty" (VN).

The HN surprise type includes products that seem familiar to the perceiver at first glance, but have unexpected tactual properties. Because the product looks familiar, the perceiver is quite certain about how the product will feel. A surprise is elicited when the apparent familiarity is proven wrong by touching the product, disconfirming the expectation. To give one example, the Flex Lamp designed by Sam Hecht (Figure 1) uses the strategy of using a new material that looks like a familiar material. His lamp looks like it is made out of matt glass (a familiar material for lamp shades), but upon touching the lamp the user finds out that the shade is flexible (it is made out of silicone rubber).

Figure 1
Flex Lamp (silicone rubber) designed by Sam Hecht, produced by Droog Design. Photograph courtesy of the designer. © Industrial Facility

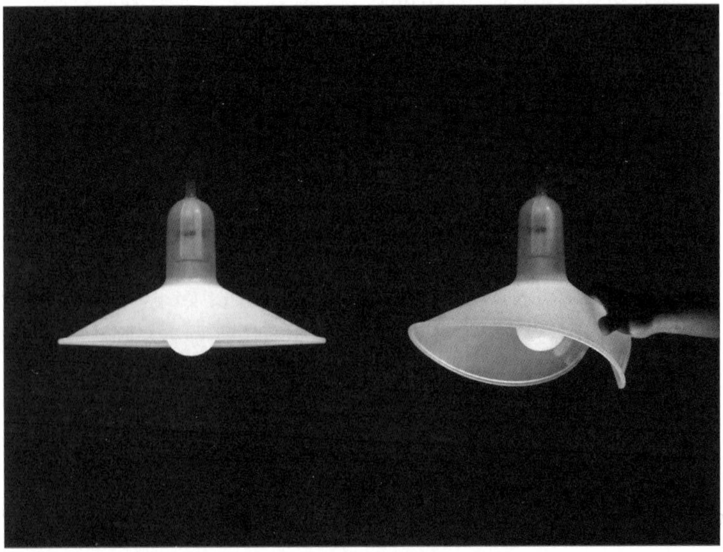

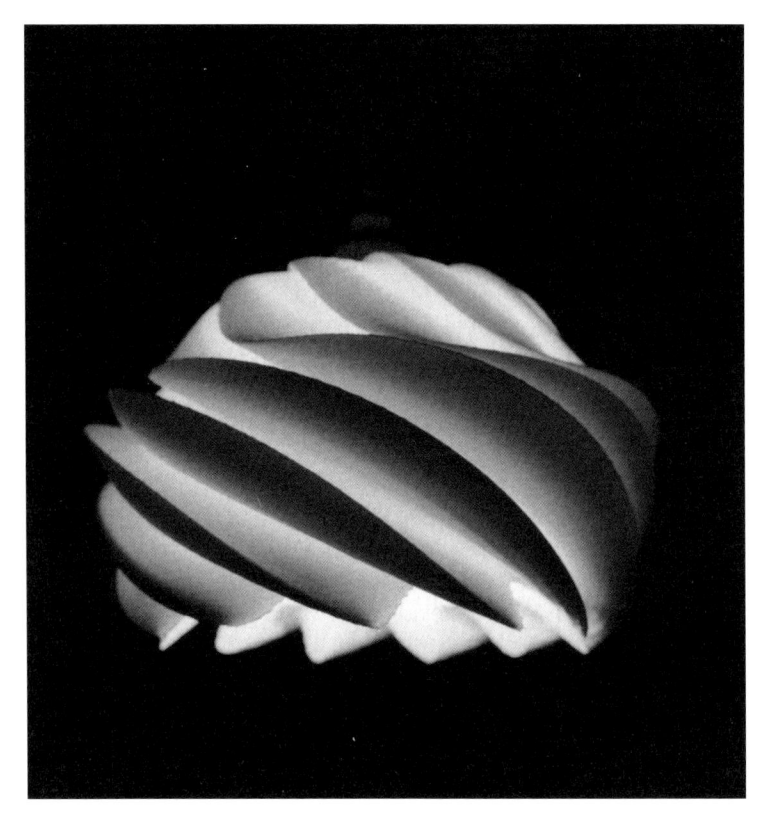

Figure 2
Lamp Konko (polyamide), designed by Willeke Evenhuis & Alex Gabriel. Photograph courtesy of the designers.

The VN type of surprise consists of products that look unfamiliar to the perceiver. Consequently, the perceiver can only form uncertain expectations about how the product will feel, based on its resemblances to other products in, for example, material or shape. A surprise is experienced whenever the uncertain expectation is disconfirmed. An example of a VN product is the lamp Konko designed by Willeke Evenhuis and Alex Gabriel (Figure 2). This lamp has an unfamiliar shape and a texture that resembles folded cloth or paper. Someone perceiving this lamp may expect it to feel light, soft and flexible. In actual fact, the lamp is made using a 3D printing technique and it feels heavy, rough and not flexible.

Several studies (Ludden et al. n.d.) have shown that people's reactions to the two types of surprising products differ. Surprise ratings were higher, and people tended to use more facial and vocal expressions of surprise, for HN than for VN products. On the other hand, people tended to use more exploratory behavior while interacting with VN products. Possibly, people enjoyed exploring VN products more than HN products, or they were more curious about the exact material properties of the VN products because they did not immediately understand exactly how their surprise reaction was brought about. In contrast, it seems as if the surprise people experienced upon touching the HN products was understood immediately, making further cognitive effort and exploration of the product unnecessary.

To conclude, consumers' comments during focus groups as well as results from empirical studies suggest that creating surprises in products can be both beneficial and harmful. It seems that for certain products, depending on the context in which the product is used, evoking surprise by creating sensory incongruity can be an effective strategy to design more interesting or amusing products. It is important to stress that the influence of the incongruity on the product's functionality should be negligible and that some forms of incongruity seem more successful than others. Provided that sensory incongruity is applied appropriately, evoking surprise in this way may be a means to create more pleasurable product experiences.

Acknowledgements

This research was supported by MAGW VIDI grant number 452-02-028 of the Netherlands Organization for Scientific Research (NWO) awarded to H.N.J. Schifferstein.

References

de Lucchi, M. and Hudson, J. 2001. *The International Design Yearbook 16*. New York: Abbeville.

Derbaix, C.and Vanhamme, J. 2003. "Inducing word-of-mouth by eliciting surprise - a pilot investigation." *Journal of Economic Psychology*, 24(1), 99–116.

Jones, B. and O'Neil, S. 1985. "Combining vision and touch in texture perception." *Perception & Psychophysics*, 37, 66–72.

Lindgreen, A. and Vanhamme, J. 2003. "To surprise or not surprise your customers: the use of surprise as a marketing tool." *Journal of Customer Behavior*, 219–42.

Lovegrove, R. and Hudson, J. 2002. *The International Design Yearbook 17*. Amsterdam: BIS.

Ludden, G.D.S. and Schifferstein, H.N.J. [n.d.] "Effects of Visual–Auditory Incongruity on Product Expression and Surprise." *Submitted*.

Ludden, G.D.S. and Schifferstein, H.N.J. [n.d.[2]] "Should Mary Smell Like Biscuit? Scent in Product Design." *Manuscript in preparation*.

Ludden, G.D.S., Schifferstein, H.N.J. and Hekkert, P. 2006. "Sensory Incongruity: Comparing Vision to Touch, Audition and Olfaction." Paper presented at the 5th Conference on Design & Emotion, Göteborg, Sweden, September 27–9.

Ludden, G.D.S., Schifferstein, H.N.J. and Hekkert, P. 2007. "Surprise as a Design Strategy." *Design Issues*, in press.

Ludden, G.D.S., Schifferstein, H.N.J. and Hekkert, P. [n.d.]. Visual–Tactual Incongruities in Products as Sources of Surprise. Submitted.

MacDonald, A.S. 2001. "Aesthetic Intelligence: Optimizing User-Centred Design." *Journal of Engineering Design*, 12(1), 37–45.

Maurer, I. and Andrew, S. 2000. *The International Design Yearbook 15*. New York: Abbeville.

Morrison, J., Horsham, M. and Hudson, J. 1999. *The International Design Yearbook 14*. London: King.

Rashid, K. 2003. *The International Design Yearbook 18*. London: King.

Schifferstein, H.N.J. and Cleiren, M.P.H.D. 2005. "Capturing Product Experiences: A Split-Modality Approach."*Acta Psychologica*, 118, 293–318.

Verbücken, M. 2003. "Towards a New Sensoriality." In E. Aarts and S. Marzano (eds), *The New Everyday: Views on Ambient Intelligence*. Rotterdam: 010 Publishers.

Sensory Design

Material Experience: Peter Zumthor's Thermal Bath at Vals

Scott Murray

Scott Murray is an architect and assistant professor in the School of Architecture, University of Illinois, Urbana-Champaign.
scmurray@uiuc.edu

Although most of his buildings are located in his native Switzerland, the architect Peter Zumthor has achieved international recognition for his work. He won the prestigious Carlsberg Architecture Prize in 1998, and his work continues to be covered widely by the international architectural press. Unlike some of his well-known contemporaries, Zumthor's oeuvre is not characterized by a signature style. Rather, each project represents an opportunity for the architect to explore the circumstances particular to each building – its site, its intended use – and to design a sensory experience that is both inventive and appropriate. In each of Zumthor's buildings, which often display exquisite minimalist detailing, one can sense the importance of architectural materials such as concrete, wood, glass and stone, in shaping the interaction between the building and its occupants. In fact, it is this dual fascination with materials and a person's direct sensory experience of architecture that defines Zumthor's approach to design. He writes that "all design work starts from the premise of this physical, objective sensuousness of architecture, of its materials. To experience architecture in a concrete way means to touch, see, hear, and smell it" (Zumthor 2006: 66).

One of Zumthor's buildings – *Therme Vals* (the Thermal Bath at Vals, Switzerland) – is particularly notable for its use of materials and attention to sensory experience. Completed in 1996, the building is located in a small farming village on a steep hillside site 1,200 m above sea level, adjacent to natural hot springs which have been utilized for therapeutic bathing since the late nineteenth century. The building, which is connected to an existing 1960s hotel complex, contains pools of various temperatures and sizes, as well as changing rooms, steam baths, indoor and outdoor lounge areas and spa treatment rooms. On a typical day, visitors may include "archi-tourists," drawn from around the world to Zumthor's famous masterpiece, as well as local residents, for whom a percentage of each day's available tickets are reserved.[1]

When one visits the building, arriving after an hour-long drive that winds through the mountains from the city of Chur, the architecture does not immediately announce itself from the exterior. This is partly because of trees planted between the village's main road and the building, but is primarily the result of Zumthor's decision to engage the building with the land such that it is built partially underground. Covered by a planted roof of wild grasses that appears as an extension of the hillside above, the new facility is almost invisible when viewed from the hotel. This is the first clue that in this design,

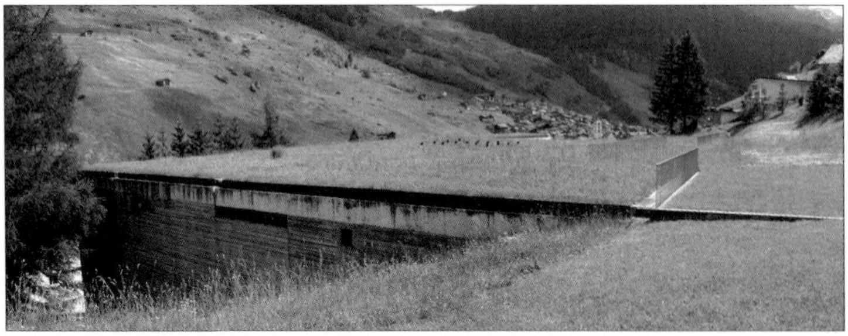

Figure 1
Exterior view of building showing planted roof and surrounding context. 2006. Photograph © Scott Murray.

Zumthor subverts the notion of architecture as a primarily visual medium – an object to be seen – in favor of a multisensory approach, creating a series of experiences revealed to the individual through use in space and time.

The dominant materials of Zumthor's building are stone and water. The stone, in conjunction with concrete, forms most of the wall and floor surfaces both inside and out; it is a bluish-gray gneiss (similar to granite) quarried from the mountains nearby.[2] The water comes from the on-site natural hot springs and is used to form pools for bathing, as well as to create other experiences of sound, smell and taste throughout. Although water is not often thought of as a building material (except as an amenity running through plumbing hidden in walls), here it is integral to the architecture. Zumthor's design exploits the symbolic significance of water, which Ivan Illich calls "the fluid that drenches the inner and outer spaces of the imagination" (Illich 1985: 24). Here, spring water is channeled and collected in various ways to enable the visitor's direct interaction with and contemplation of it. It is this unique combination of two materials extracted from the surrounding mountains – stone and water – which forms the architecture, inextricably ties the building to its site and, in a sense, mediates between the visitor and the specificity of the place, its history and geology. Zumthor articulates this relationship, writing of his project for Vals: "Mountain, stone, water, building in stone, building with stone, building into the mountain, building out of the mountain – our attempts to give this chain of words an architectural interpretation, to translate into architecture its meaning and sensuousness, guided our design for the building and step by step gave it form" (Zumthor 1998: 138).

The entry sequence to the thermal bath begins in the lobby of the hotel. One descends from there to a lower level, walking through a dark, subterranean passage to reach the entry hall of the baths. Underground, devoid of natural light and surrounded by stone, this hall has the feel of a dark cave, albeit a cave notable for its right angles and refined modernist detailing. The sound of trickling spring water emanates from a series of bronze faucets along the right-hand wall, designed as drinking fountains to give visitors their first introduction (literally their first taste) of the water as it springs from the earth behind the wall. To the left, a series of openings lead to changing rooms, also dimly lit. Passing through doors on the other side of the changing rooms, one arrives on a platform raised above the main floor of the baths, from which the main pool is visible, along with glimpses of the landscape beyond through large glazed openings in the far wall. Very narrow, linear skylights sliced through the roof above bring in controlled natural light, which dramatically grazes the uneven surface of the stone walls. A long processional ramp leads down to the main level, where one may begin to explore the layout of the baths.

This main space of the building contains one large pool with 32° C water, around and within which several large stone-clad volumes are arranged. Upon exploration, one finds an opening into each volume that leads to a room-sized space within, each designed for a different sensory experience and marked by a sense of discovery. These spaces have the feel of being carved out of a block of solid stone, just as the building itself seems to be carved out of the mountain. One volume contains the *fire bath* (42° C) while another is the *ice bath* (12° C). The *flower bath* contains 30° C water the surface of which is covered with floating flower petals, creating an intense aroma and tactile experience. One volume contains a well from which spring water can be tasted, while yet another is a completely dark space called the *sounding stone*, with benches and

Scott Murray

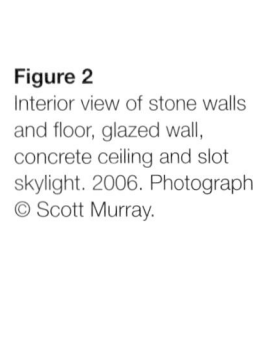

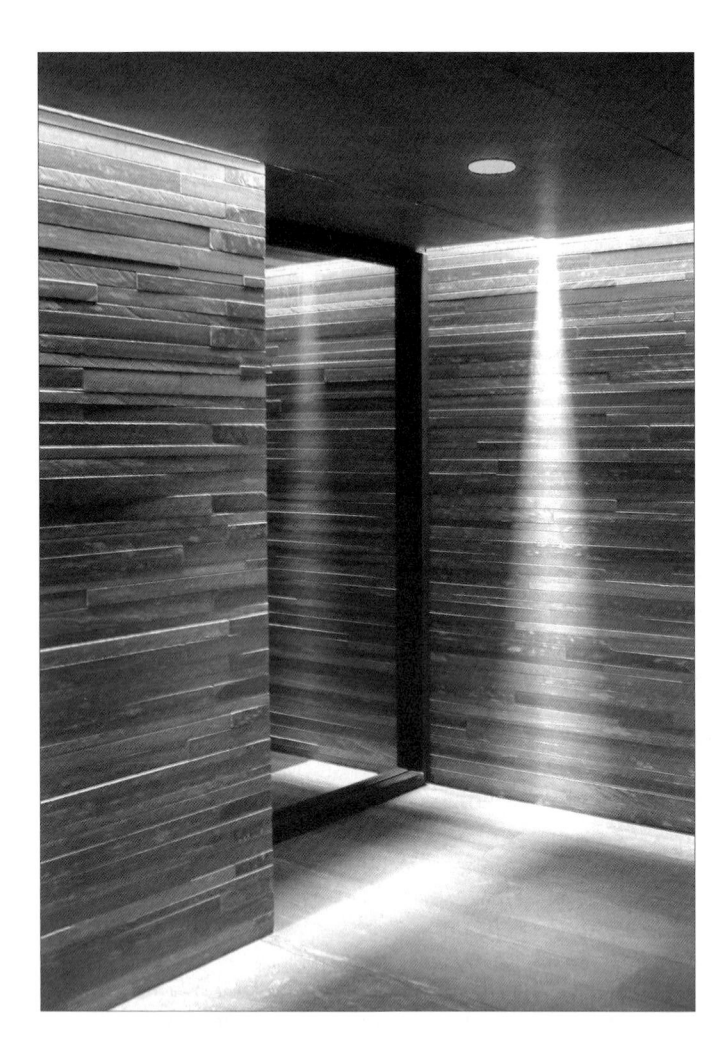

Figure 2
Interior view of stone walls and floor, glazed wall, concrete ceiling and slot skylight. 2006. Photograph © Scott Murray.

hidden speakers through which recorded sound art by composer Fritz Hauser is played.

There is no predetermined sequence for experiencing these spaces. Visitors are free to make their own path into and among the various pools and spaces at their own pace and in their own order, resulting in a multiplicity of circulation routes and constant activity. Haptic and auditory encounters prevail: the enveloping of the body in spring water of varying temperatures; the rhythmic sound of bare feet walking on wet stone; echoes of voices and splashing water, louder in the large central space contrasting with quiet solitude in the smaller baths. Elements to be gripped by the hand, such as door pulls and handrails, are all made of bronze, their smooth texture and warm color tone a counterpoint to the ever-present stone. One of the most interesting experiences occurs where an inside pool connects directly to the outside pool through an opening in the large glass wall that divides the two. Here one can move from inside to outside while submerged in water, as if swimming out of a cave. Outside are stone terraces for relaxation, where emerging from the pool, one encounters a reawakening to the alpine climate as wet skin meets crisp, cool air, tempered by the warmth of direct sunlight.

Any built work of architecture can be read as a study of the materials used in its construction. In the process of design, such materials are typically evaluated for their structural properties, their aesthetic appearance and their suitability in relation to a variety of functional performance criteria. But in some cases, the materials of the building contribute more than mere functionality. As the physical embodiment of the ideas behind a design, materials can take on conceptual importance. Zumthor suggests that in the end, the direct experience of the materials may even surpass the idea. "Material is stronger than idea," says Zumthor, "it's stronger than an image because it's really there, and it's there in its own right" (Spier 2001: 19). Zumthor's Thermal Bath at Vals is an exemplary building in which the selection, deployment and detailing of architectural materials, particularly stone and water, are as important as form-making or the shaping of space and are in fact integral to one's experience of the architecture.

Notes

1. The village of Vals served as Zumthor's client for the design and paid for the construction of the Bath. Reflecting on the difficulties of achieving the construction of such a unique design and the important role of the client in the building process, Zumthor credits the villagers for their progressive architectural sensibility and their desire "to do something special, not something usual, a bath like everybody has" (Spier 2001: 22).
2. The walls of the building are primarily a load-bearing composite of natural gneiss stone and site-cast concrete, which Zumthor refers to as "poured stone" (Spier 2001: 18). For details of the wall assembly, see Zumthor 2001:170–2. To achieve a variety of desired effects throughout the building, Zumthor specified a number of different surface treatments for the gneiss, ranging from "polished, sandpaper grading 550, to sawn, chiseled, and the way it comes out of the quarry – split" (Spier 2001:19). In this way, the material is fine-tuned to suit specific applications.

References

Illich, Ivan. 1985. *H_2O and the Waters of Forgetfulness*. Berkeley: Heyday Books.

Spier, Steven. 2001. "Place, Authorship and the Concrete: Three Conversations with Peter Zumthor," *ARQ Architectural Research Quarterly*, 5 (1) 15–31.

Zumthor, Peter. 1998. *Architecture and Urbanism February 1998 Extra Edition*. Tokyo: a+u Publishing Co., Ltd.

——. 2006. *Thinking Architecture*. Basel: Birkhauser.

BOOK REVIEWS

Cottage in a Boudoir

Sensation and Sensibility: Viewing Gainsborough's Cottage Door, by Ann Bermingham, ed.

New Haven, CT: Yale University Press, 2005, 208 pages. ISBN-10: 0300110022. $65.00.

Jessica Riskin

Author of *Science in the Age of Sensibility: The Sentimental Empiricists of the French Enlightenment*, Jessica Riskin teaches in the History Department at Stanford University. She is writing a book on the body-machine from Descartes to Darwin.
jriskin@stanford.edu

One day in 1344 or 1345, the Sienese painter, Ambrogio Lorenzetti, must have had a momentous idea: it occurred to him that he could paint a boat. He did so. The boat sits at the edge of a small lake. There is a castle on the shore, a field and several trees. The painting is called *Un castello in riva a un lago* (*Castle by a Lakeshore*). Around the same time, Lorenzetti also painted a city overlooking the ocean and called it *Una città vicino al mare* (*City by the Sea*). The two paintings hang with understated drama in the *Pinacoteca nazionale* in Siena, amidst a blizzard of images of saints and angels, the Annunciation, the Madonna and Child, the Adoration of the Magi, the Coronation of the Virgin, the Death of the Virgin, the Assumption of the Virgin, Christ on the Cross, the Passion. Making one's way among the crucifixions and nativities, the martyrs, the allegories of humility, suffering, faith and redemption, one comes abruptly upon a small boat, some scrubby trees, a seaside town. To see them there is a reverse-epiphany, a sudden discovery of the secular. A realization, one realizes, was required to make these paintings. At a given moment, Lorenzetti must have thought, "I could just paint a boat." He may have lived to regret it: three or four years afterward, he died of the plague.

When Thomas Gainsborough painted his *Cottage Door* about four-and-a-half centuries later (c. 1780), it required an equivalent imaginative shift. As Ann Bermingham explains in her Introduction to *Sensation and Sensibility: Viewing Gainsborough's* Cottage Door, Gainsborough was the first British artist to fix his attention upon cottages and cottage life, subjects which, before him, had fallen "below the period's threshold of visibility, not so much ignored as not seen" (p.1) The book, which Bermingham edited, is the impressive catalog of a 2005 exhibit of which she was curator, jointly undertaken by The Huntington and the Yale Center for British Art, centering upon Gainsborough's painting and his other representations of cottages and their inhabitants.

As the catalog essays richly delineate, the imaginative shift involved in focusing a painting upon a cottage door was manifold, taking place not only on the level of subject matter, but also of style, technique and philosophy. The works in the exhibit were among the first British visual expressions of the cultural movement devoted to what its participants understood as "sensibility": an inextricable fusion of moral and emotional sentiment and physical sensation. Eighteenth-century sensibilists took a defining interest in the mechanisms of sensation and in the sciences that studied these. But their attention to scientific and technical matters was traditionally underplayed by later generations of historians who assumed a disjunction between science and sentiment. A particular strength of *Sensation and Sensibility* is that it recovers the inseparability, in the eyes of Gainsborough and his contemporaries, of moral and emotional from physiological and physical questions.

Nursing is the opening example: Gainsborough's cottages are commonly graced by women nursing babies. Susan Sloman explains in the book's first essay that these figures reflected a mid-century vogue for natural child-rearing. A similar fusion of physiology and morals occurred in the physician George Cheyne's theory of the benefits of horseback riding, "variously twitching the Nervous Fibres, to brace and contract them, as new Scenes amuse the mind" (p. 41). Cheyne's regimen sent Gainsborough out into the countryside each day and these rides, Sloman suggests, during which Gainsborough's optical fibers and moral faculty alike were tweaked by glimpses of cottage life, probably inspired his paintings of the subject.

Making a slogan of nature, as distinct from social artifice, the sensibilists dwelled on the tension between the two. As Bermingham points out in her introductory essay, Gainsborough's cottages, covered in foliage, seem to have grown directly out of the landscape.

The politics of these renditions of peasant society as organic, a kind of not-society, are the subject of both John Barrell's and Michael Rosenthal's essays. Barrell argues that a sometimes subliminal class politics shaped Gainsborough's and others' representations of cottages and cottagers. In particular, an ideal of rural poverty was at work in Gainsborough's depictions of peasants as they appeared in his cottage scenes: "remote from society … entirely focused on the family" (p.54), in short, reassuringly disunited, engaging in no kind of collective endeavor. Along similar lines, Rosenthal examines the contrasting implications of history painting, associated through its subjects with commerce and republicanism, and landscape painting. Gainsborough's landscapes, offered in part as challenges to traditional history paintings, emerge in this context as essentially conservative, reactions against the developing agrarian capitalism and the specter of republicanism.

One expression of their overarching interest in the tensions between nature and artifice was sensibilists' alertness to the artifice of their own work. Amal Asfour and Paul Williamson argue that Gainsborough responded to a growing preoccupation among his contemporaries with the disjunction between actual visual experience and its artistic representation by embracing the artificiality of his painted images. He imbued these, Asfour and Williamson write, with a "radical sense of [idyllic] unreality" (pp.97–8). Designing his later landscapes in characteristically curving lines, Gainsborough also seemed to situate his observer "within the world of the image," a perspective which, together with the feeling of unreality, constituted "an appeal to the viewer's imagination" (p.105). Gainsborough thus assumed, Asfour and Williamson suggest, a new activity on the part of the spectator, not the objective observation of the "lordly Rubensian eye" but an act of "subjective, sensible imagination" (p.108).

The settings in which sensibilist paintings were displayed also highlighted the contrast between the natural world of the painting and the highly artificial world of the viewer. As Dongho Chun's and Ann Bermingham's essays delineate, *The Cottage Door* achieved the pinnacle of its reputation on display in Sir John Leicester's "tent room." Leicester, an influential patron and private collector, acquired the painting in 1809 and kept it until his death in 1827. His "tent room" was a converted boudoir on the first floor of his gallery in a London townhouse at 24 Hill Street. The room had a striped, tented ceiling of blue and white calico; its windows and walls were covered in fluted drapes of crimson moreen; oil lamps provided the lighting; the gold-tasseled yellow valances had crimson rosettes and crosses; and there were mirrors on all sides. This richly upholstered setting, Bermingham observes, made an incongruous context for *The Cottage Door*. Yet that very incongruity, it appears from her own and her collaborators' discussions, in fact helped to dramatize Gainsborough's point. The rustic simplicity of the world within the painting appeared silhouetted against the lavish opulence of the room it occupied.

The tent room's important role in shaping the fortunes of *The Cottage Door* was consistent with the artist's own keen awareness, while designing his paintings, of the process of perception that would come at the other end, when viewers arrived before the finished work, and of its subjective, manipulable nature. Gainsborough's characteristic, loose brushwork, William Vaughan observes in the book's penultimate chapter, meant that a "normal viewing-distance," rather than a position right up close to the canvas, constituted the point at which "separately perceived brushstrokes suddenly combine in the mind to form an image" (p.168). As a result, Vaughan suggests, Gainsborough incorporated a consciousness of the "magical" aspect of painting, conjuring a world out of patches of color, into the experience of viewing his work.

An abiding interest in techniques for manipulating the process of perception – the magic lantern, the *camera obscura*, tricks with mirrors and lighting – crucially informed Gainsborough's paintings. Thus, the essays of the final section situate these with regard to the overlapping traditions of natural magic and popular science. In particular, Vaughan and Iain McCalman, in the closing essay, discuss the inspiration that Gainsborough derived from the "Eidophusikon," the mechanical theater built by his friend, the Strasbourg landscape artist and set-designer, Philippe Jacques de Loutherbourg.

The Eidophusikon, which caused a sensation when it was first exhibited in London in 1781, incorporated "hidden lighting, magic lantern slides, colored silk filters, clockwork automata, three-dimensional models, painted transparencies, and a sophisticated sound system" (p.181) to enact five scenes: dawn on the Thames; Gibraltar at noon; a sunset over the Bay of Naples; a moonrise over the Mediterranean; a storm wrecking a ship at sea. The following year, an updated version included Niagara Falls; a waterspout off the Japanese coast; a naval spectacle at Plymouth with tiny, automaton sailors; and Milton's Pandemonium. The Eidophusikon, along with the magic lantern and *camera obscura*, plainly informed Gainsborough's "showbox," a closed, wooden box into which a viewer could peer to see a landscape glowing in the darkness. Gainsborough painted the landscapes for the showbox on glass slides; spectators saw them illuminated from behind and magnified by a lens in the showbox's viewing window.

To return, for a moment, to Lorenzetti's *Un castello in riva a un lago*, it was of course about a castle by a lake with a little boat, but it also – precisely by being about those things – constituted a shift of artistic attention from the object of the painting to the process of representation itself. Similarly, *Sense and Sensibility* shows that Gainsborough's cottage doors were not just about cottage doors and cottage life, but also about tent rooms and intricate machinery, the devices of experimental physics and the laws of optics. A celebration of simplicity, nature and a simple, natural way of life characterized the most directly visible aspect of Gainsborough's cottage door paintings, namely, their subject matter, but that was only one of their defining elements. Counterbalancing the naturalness of the content was the self-conscious artifice of the execution and presentation, informed by the artist's deep interest in the malleability of perception. The authors of *Sensation and Sensibility* eloquently demonstrate that the style of sensibility did not express a single impulse, but rather two opposing preoccupations. The natural world within the representations took shape against the artist's depiction of his own domain as thoroughly artificial.

The Taste Culture Reader

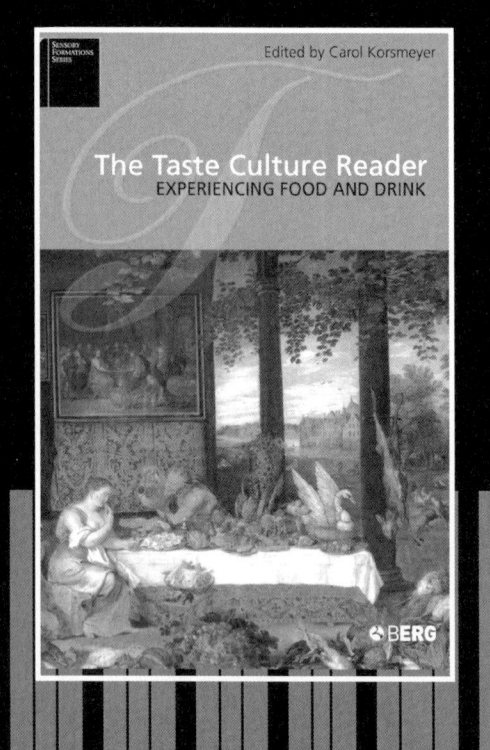

Experiencing Food and Drink

Edited by Carolyn Korsmeyer

384pp • 234 x 156 mm
PB 978 1 84520 061 9 £19.99 • $34.95
HB 978 1 84520 060 2 £55.00 • $105.00

The Taste Culture Reader is part of the **SENSORY FORMATIONS** series, edited by David Howes. Other books in the series include *Empire of the Senses*, *The Auditory Culture Reader*, *The Book of Touch*, and *The Smell Culture Reader*. All are available to order online at www.bergpublishers.com.

BERG

From Eve's apple to Proust's madeleine to today's culinary tourism, food looms large in culture. Sociologists and anthropologists study cooking and eating practices across the globe. Debates about health and nutrition are common in news reports. Yet despite its fundamental relationship to food, taste is mysteriously absent from most of these discussions. The flavours of foods permeate social relations, religious and other occasions. Charged with memory, emotion, desire and aversion, taste is arguably the most evocative of the senses. *The Taste Culture Reader* explores the sensuous dimensions of eating and drinking, from the physiology of the tongue to the embodiment of social identities and enactment of ceremonial meanings. A cornucopia of historical, cross-cultural and theoretical views is offered, drawing from anthropology, sociology, history, philosophy, science – and more. This book will interest anyone seeking to understand more fully the importance of food and flavor in human experience.

Rich Pickings: Cultures and Histories of Taste

The Taste Culture Reader: Experiencing Food and Drink, by Carolyn Korsmeyer (ed.)

Oxford and New York: Berg, 2005, 421 pages. PB 1-84520-061-9. £19.99

Taste: A Literary History, by Denise Gigante

New Haven and London: Yale University Press, 2005, 241 pages. Cloth 0-300-10652-1. £20.00

Jean Duruz

Jean Duruz is a Senior Lecturer in cultural studies, School of Communication, University of South Australia.
jean.duruz@unisa.edu.au

My own dinner party piece, which has prompted writing elsewhere (Duruz, forthcoming) draws on the memory of a dreary winter I spent in England. This is a tale of Australian yearning for one of our most popular national dishes – the Straits Chinese dish, *laksa*, with its tastes of coconut milk, chilli, galangal and lemongrass lingering on the tongue. The evocative presence of this dish from a borrowed foodway, haunting the culinary landscapes of England, my ancestral home, continues to surprise me. More importantly, however, this fragment of remembering underlines the often unrecognized significance of taste itself: taste as deeply embodied cultural knowledge which resonates in everyday life, and sometimes, in unexpected ways. Recent analytical writing on taste (and smell, its close relative) should have much to offer in regard to the poignancy of "tasted" experience or the potential of the disruptive moment. In this respect, Carolyn Korsmeyer's edited collection, *The Taste Culture Reader: Experiencing Food and Drink*, and Denise Gigante's account of gastronomy and British Romanticism, *Taste: A Literary History*, both set satisfying, though very different, tables for intellectual consumption.

Prompted by this everyday drift to *laksa* dreaming, I set out to trawl *The Taste Culture Reader*. The task at first seems daunting. Ambitious in scope and working "against the grain" of traditional (Kantian) privileging of vision and hearing in hierarchies of the senses, this collection of thirty-seven contributions allows taste a critical, embodied presence – one that is complex, nuanced and redolent with possibility. The selection of writing represents a wide range of disciplines and genres – medicine, psychology, gastronomy, oenology, anthropology, sociology, philosophy, religious studies, cultural geography, cultural studies, history, literary studies, biography; the extracts map locations as diverse as cheese shops in the Netherlands (Watson), a Carib-Northumbria restaurant on the moors of Northumberland (James), cemeteries in rural Mexico during Dias de Muertos [Days of the Dead] (Carmichael and Sayer) and impoverished farms in a high valley of the Ecuadorian Andes (Weismantel); the collection moves back in time (see Schivelbusch on the spice trade, for example), in memory (there is a rich collection of writing here) and forward to "postmodern" concerns in relation to "artificial" tastes and smells (Classen, Howes and Synnot), "authentic," "simulated" and "hybrid" foods (James; Haden; Heldke) and the nostalgic tastes of nation and their re-invention through performance (Goldstein).

A formidable array of established writers is included in the collection. These range from those gastronomic and philosophical 'gods' – Brillat-Savarin, Hume, Kant and, of course, Proust – to familiar "names" in the present, such as Goody, Mintz, Mennell, Gabaccia and Visser. The collection also casts its political/theoretical net widely. Korsmeyer's introductory comments stake a claim on relations of class, ethnicity, gender and sexuality, though of these, class – a dominant thread in discussions of "high" and "low" cuisine and Bourdieu's account of the "luxury/necessity" distinction – has a more explicit presence within the book's conceptual frameworks. In contrast, other dimensions of difference tend to be more subtly embedded in the details of case studies. (Curiously, at least in the book's Introduction, we find "sexuality" elided into "sexual behavior" and, even then, this is rapidly relegated to a back seat, as a subset of gender relations. [p. 49])

A nagging question, however: is this collection too diffuse with too many competing "tastes" to constitute satisfying reading? To be fair, this is a problem endemic to the genre. The challenge for such anthologies is to achieve a sense of wholeness, however disparate their elements might seem. The organization of this volume, with its thematic sections (for example, "Body and Soul" [taste and religion], "Eloquent Flavors" [specific tastes – salt, sugar, spices]) and notes summarizing each section, certainly implies specific territories to be covered and logical routes through these. On the other hand, it is not simply a case of writing a "collection" into being but also a question of readers' appetites and consumption practices. Here I am suggesting that just as one might doggedly follow the set menu for this feast, there are other ways to eat at the table. My own preference here is for a *dégustation* – a range of small dishes chosen for their individual "tastes," yet ordered with an eye to complementary flavors.

On this occasion, my *dégustation* might include Paul Stoller and Cheryl Olkes' "repulsive"sauce, eaten while on fieldwork with the Songhay in Nigeria – a mundane instance of cultural life and interaction which, viewed differently, disrupts the analytic taken-for-granted, in powerful ways. Perversely, this sauce, deliberately flavored with anger and intended insult, confirms the guests' membership in the community. The end-result of this curious ethnographic moment is a finely-textured analysis – thoughtful, imaginative, ironic – and conscious of its own sensory potential (the repetitive rhythms of "a thin sauce for a thick social occasion," for example) (pp. 133–41).

There are many other moments to tempt, though space is limited here: David Sutton's intriguing "'The prickly pear today, it was honey'" (p. 313) drawn from his fieldwork on the Greek island of Kalymnos, or Lisa Heldke's meditation on her own first contact with "galangal," or "Thai ginger," or Alison James' reflections on culinary hybridity (beware the Chinese pizza or "dumbed down" Indian dish, depleted of quantities of chilli and ghee), or Nadia Seremetakis' peach, a variety known as "the breast of Aphrodite." Like other tastes haunting this book, the memory of this no-longer-available peach is not simply an instance of poetic remembering; instead, the peach continues, throughout the chapter, as a phenomenological space in which public culture is understood and played out ("the object invested with sensory memory speaks") (p. 303). Meanwhile, the argument of ghostly absences is taken even further by Classen, Howes and Synnott's chapter ("Artificial Flavours"). This chapter describes an far more worrying scenario than "inauthentic" Chinese pizza or even re-located *laksa*: this is a future in which culinary imperialism is the theft of the materiality of food itself, and only its simulated smells linger, floating free of their referents.

If *The Taste Culture Reader* offers diverse and beguiling postmodern moments of edible writing, Denise Gigante's *Taste: A Literary History* presents a formal banquet. The pace is measured, the argument dense with scholarly references, the structure a sequence of courses that traverses the gastronomic terrains of eighteenth- and nineteenth-century British Romanticism. Together, the chapters accumulate an elegant narrative, though (as the last chapter, "The Gastronome and the Snob: George IV," indicates) not necessarily one of "progress" in an enlightenment or modernist sense. Instead, the text traces in poetry, essays, philosophical and other writing a series of consuming figures: the Man of Taste, the Romantic Gourmand, gutsy urban flesh-eaters, vampiric cannibals/capitalists, melancholic/existential yearners...

For entrée – if the reader follows the menu – Gigante teases out the "complex relations between aesthetic taste and the more substantial phenomenon of appetite" (p. 3). *Taste*'s main courses consist of chapters on Milton, the "taste philosophers" (Shaftesbury, Addison, Hume and Burke), Wordsworth, Lamb, Byron and Keats all engaging with the tangled histories of Romantic aesthetics and the rise of consumer societies. For dessert, Gigante examines middle-class dinner parties and the figure of the dandy during the Victorian era (think Jos Sedley in Thackeray's *Vanity Fair* as parody of George IV or the dinner parties described by Dickens in *Our Mutual Friend*). In these Victorian novels, says Gigante, dinners and dandies perform as snobbish displays of consumer "style"; this is "taste" without taste ("they don't even know that they don't know") (p. 180).

Obviously, for a student of British Romanticism, this book has much to offer. However, for my preoccupation with meanings of the everyday and their sensory geographies and histories, the originality of *Taste: A Literary History* lies in its complex archaeology of the conceptual connectedness of aesthetics and appetite in contrast to their more usual positioning in opposition. Interestingly and compellingly, the argument examines porosities of boundaries between popular culture and "high" art, gustatory and aesthetic pleasures, the metaphorical and the embodied. The chapter on Wordsworth provides a case in point.

Adopting the poet's own metaphor of "feeding" as the chapter's leitmotif, Gigante builds a skilful account of how transcendental relations with the natural world become intense and visceral forms of consumption. In Wordsworth's own imagery, the Romantic poet literally "feeds" on the landscape. At the same time, however, Wordsworth distances himself from, again in his own words, the "noisy" pleasures of mass culture ("a pantomime, a farce, or a puppet-show") and the "molestation of cheap trains pouring out their hundreds at a time along the margins of Windermere" (p. 79). Obviously, this (snobbish) distinction – between the greedy, despoiling masses from "cheap trains" and the intellectual and spiritual purity of the "Romantic Gourmand's" attachment to his beloved lakes – poses no contradiction for Wordsworth, and is hardly surprising for the reader: it is the classic dilemma of the "sensitive" tourist who seeks "authenticity." Gigante's argument, however, is more complicated. She draws together these seemingly opposing meanings of "taste" to show how each "feeds"/ "feeds" on/off the other in a symbiotic relationship. Here, those distinctions between aesthetics and appetite really begin to unravel: Wordsworth's sublime "feeding," in fact encouraged mass tourism of the "picturesque"; contradictorily, his solitary longing contributed to a collective romance that, in turn, cluttered his horizons with consuming others. Furthermore, Wordsworth himself became a toured landscape, as the poet received more and more "fashionable visitors" (Keats, quoted by Gigante, p. 88) to his home, with these numbering five hundred a year by the 1840s (p. 88).

For the project of sensory studies, then, it seems that both *The Taste Culture Reader* and *Taste: A Literary History* have much to offer. Crucially, they remind us of the significance of taste in cultural life, its dense symbolism, its multiplicity of meanings. Taste in both of these volumes refuses the ground of pure aesthetics or of bounded, single-discipline approaches to academic work. From very different perspectives, both of these books offer a trail of rich pickings – creative reflections on embodied cultures of consumption … how we eat and drink together, how we remember and forget, how we write about this and, finally, how we imagine we might live.

Reference

Duruz, Jean. n.d. "From Malacca to Adelaide: Fragments towards a Biography of Cooking, Yearning and *Laksa*." In Sidney C.H Cheung, Tan Chee Beng and Maria Siumi Tam (eds.), *Food and Foodways in Asia*. Richmond, Surrey: Routledge Curzon.

Exhibition and Conference Reviews

Tropicália: A Revolution in Brazilian Culture

Organized by and first exhibited at the Barbican Art Gallery, London, February 13–May 22, 2006. Curated by Carlos Basualdo. Traveling to the Bronx Museum of the Arts, New York, October 7, 2006–January 28, 2007

Jonathan Goodman

Jonathan Goodman is a writer based in New York who specializes in modern and contemporary art. He currently teaches at Pratt Institute and the Parsons School of Design.
threerooms@earthlink.net

"Tropicália: A Revolution in Brazilian Culture" is the first major, comprehensive show to document the Tropicália movement, which lasted in Brazil from 1967 to 1972, in the face of the military regime that had taken over in 1964. A brilliantly improvised counterculture was created to protest against and resist the military government; its achievements included radical new works in art, music, film, theater and architecture, with the emphasis moving always in the direction of the ephemeral and the spontaneous. While there are similarities to the American alternative culture that arose during the same period, it appears that the Tropicália era was a movement made more cohesive by the military government in Brazil, whose repression only resulted in the Brazilian arts movement

Exhibition Reviews

becoming more and more critical, both directly and indirectly, of the status quo. The name Tropicália was taken from a sharply subversive installation by the noted artist Helio Oiticica, created in 1967, as well as by the highly influential, and popular, 1968 album *Tropicália ou Panis et Circensis,* fronted by the well-known singers Gilberto Gil and Caetano Veloso. Curator Carlos Basualdo emphasizes that while Tropicália is noted primarily for its musical achievements, the show is meant to draw attention to the broad range of its accomplishments, not only in music:

> In part, this exhibition is an effort to restore the proper multi-disciplinary nature of the Tropicália movement... In the end these artists drew from a range of disciplines and local and international influences to create new hybrid forms that were uniquely Brazilian. (Basualdo 2006)

"Tropicália" comprised some 250 objects, many of which were shown in the Bronx Museum of the Art's newly built addition, where I saw the exhibition, a striking construction of glass and metal that brought light into the interior of the building. The exhibition of Brazilian art underscored the importance of the Bronx Museum to its local residents, the majority of whom are of Hispanic background. In so large a show, there was the inevitable doubling back to spaces seen earlier in one's visit; sometimes it was hard to follow the thread of thought behind the ordering of the objects, especially if the visitor did not know much about the Tropicália movement. But no matter, the sometimes confusing arrangement of art seemed, in the long run, to emphasize the pluralist, deeply democratic nature of Tropicália's intentions. With exhibits by such renowned artists as Oiticica, Lygia Clark and Lygia Pape, "Tropicália" offered viewers

Figure 1
View of "Tropicália: A Revolution in Brazilian Culture," with assume vivid astro focus's *Garden 10*, 2004, in foreground. Photograph: Norman McGrath, courtesy the Bronx Museum of the Arts.

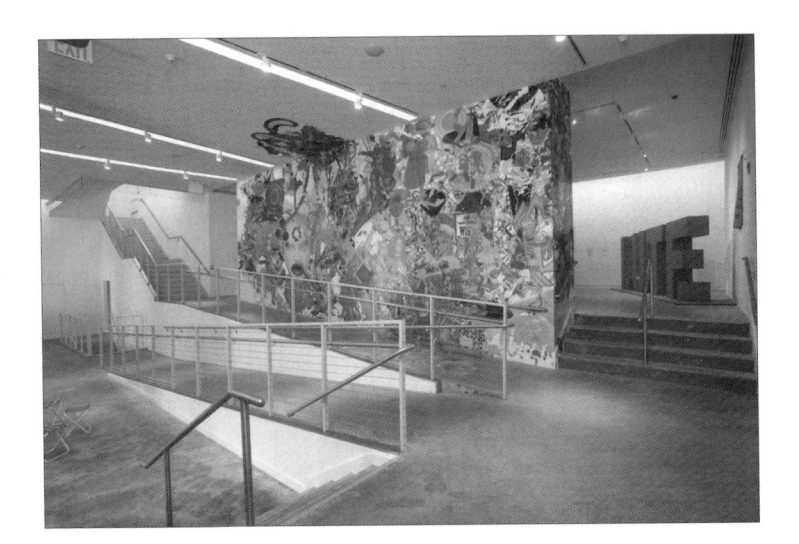

a chance to see art by major figures of the period, as well as the ephemera – books, pamphlets, fashion – by lesser-known artists of that particular moment in time. The overall sense of the show was that of a profoundly pluralistic, at times even anarchic, rush of creativity that connected deeply with the poor as well as with the relatively privileged artworld.

Oiticica's installation *Tropicália* (1967), which gave the movement its name, was the centerpiece of the exhibition. Originally shown in the 1967 exhibition "New Brazilian Objectivity," at the Museum of Modern Art in Rio de Janeiro, *Tropicália* was highly creative in its innovations. Consisting of sand and labyrinth-like walkways, the installation reproduced the sensory experience of the Brazilian slums, combining wood, plastic and corrugated steel into facsimiles of the vividly colorful homes of the poor. In the maze was a television giving only static – the perfect symbol of the increasingly popular presence of the media in people's lives – as well as two parrots, who further increased the tropical feel of the exhibit. Taken as an interactive and visceral environment, the artist's development of a vernacular architecture as an all-inclusive experience shows remarkable prescience regarding art practice in the years to come. During the late 1960s and early 1970s in America, Pop art was at its zenith, with figures like Andy Warhol celebrating the materialist pleasures of American capitalism. Oiticica's maze is far different in its implications, in its embrace of the dispossessed, whose energies he taps into so as to connect with a segment of society largely left out of the picture in art in the Americas. The environment is also, as I have said, amazingly ahead of its times in a formal sense – artists in America would not use installation and sensory immersion as a mainstream strategy until the early 1990s.

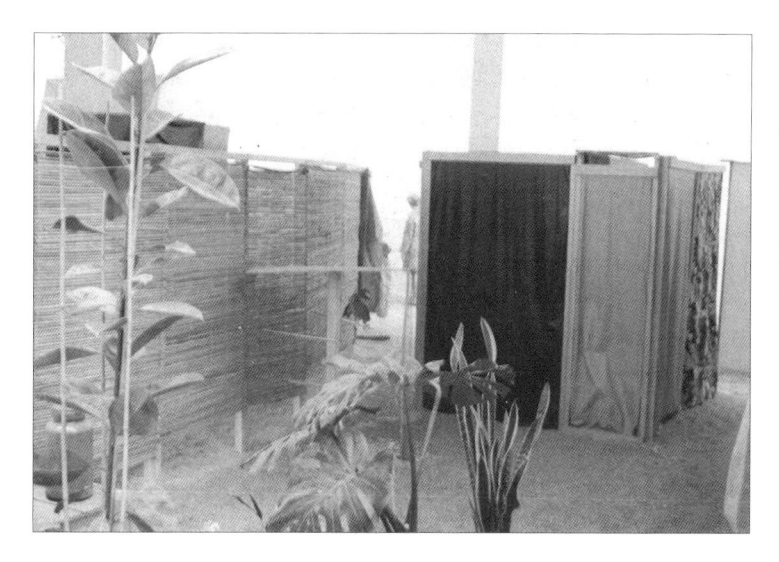

Figure 2
Hélio Oiticica, *Tropicália* (detail), 1967. Installation view at "Tropicália: A Revolution in Brazilian Culture." Copyright © Projeto Hélio Oiticica (Rio de Janeiro, Brazil). Courtesy the Bronx Museum of the Arts.

It is important to remember that the major push behind the Tropicália era was musical in nature; the thematic album *Tropicália ou Panis et Circensis*, released in 1968, became one of the most highly regarded albums of its time in Brazil. The exhibition paid attention to the music by including tracks from the album on the iPods given to visitors, who could hear Gil, Veloso, the band Os Mutantes and other influential singers, whose mixture of samba, bossa nova and rock would prove to be both popular and critically acclaimed. As it turned out, popular music became the means for expressing disaffection for the military regime in Brazil, whose practices would grow more brutal with the passage of time. One is tempted to see similar positions in contemporary art in America, but the American position did not truly address the poor, something the Tropicália artists and musicians were very careful to do. In this sense it is fair to say that the Brazilian moment was genuinely politicized, even if its ethics were being communicated by such soft signifiers as pop music.

It hardly seems fair to skip over the achievements of many talented artists in so large a show. There were capes by Oiticica that visitors could try on themselves; videos showed people dancing in the streets wearing the colorful clothing, as a way of highlighting the improvisatory nature of life in the slums. This sense of being in the moment, based upon a refusal to separate art from life, gave the Tropicália movement its air of festive opposition, in which the harsh realities of government were not so much directly attacked as they were indirectly subverted, not by a version of American flower power but by a more sophisticated feeling of spontaneous joy. Lygia Pape's small, interactive paper cutout artwork demonstrated that intimacy in art could also be conceptually demanding and visually enjoyable; her geometrical symbols – circles and arrows – resulted in images of uncommon grace. Another piece by Lygia Pape, *Wheel of Delight* (1968), highlighted sensuous confusion by having viewers taste water in bowls that had been given different colors and flavors. The disconnect between the colors and taste of the water challenged the audience to make sense of the unusual experience, which went against preconceived notions. Lygia Clark offered a marvelous *Sensorial Book* (1966/2005), in which shells, stones, rubber bands, water, metal, a mirror and steel wool were enclosed in plastic bags, presenting complex sensorial experiences to the visitors who handled them. Other interactive objects included *Sensorial Masks* (1967) made of different materials that altered visual perception through aural, olfactive and tactile sensations, as well as goggles that fell outward from their frames, away from the wearer's eyes.

More recent artists also showed in "Tropicália." The collective assume vivid astro focus presented a brightly colored wallpaper and floor decals and stickers in a heavily psychedelic style; the work, all stemming from 2004, shows that the spirit of the movement lingers, even if primarily through nostalgic interpretations. The famous singer

Gilberto Gil is now minister of culture for the Brazilian government – who would have thought that such a thing would have come to pass? One has the sense that the barriers between what has been too crudely called high and low culture are not so impermeable in Brazil, where there is the feeling of a more fluid exchange between performers and artists and their audience. At present, in the American context, the class-exacerbated problems of elite and vernacular expressiveness only underscore the extent to which American culture has succumbed to a rigidification of social placement. "Tropicália," always close to the powerfully sensory and expressive energies of the dispossessed, showed New York a thing or two about connecting with backgrounds and perceptual sensibilities too easily written off in North America.

Reference
Basualdo, Carlos. 2006. Personal communication.

The Emotions
A Cultural Reader

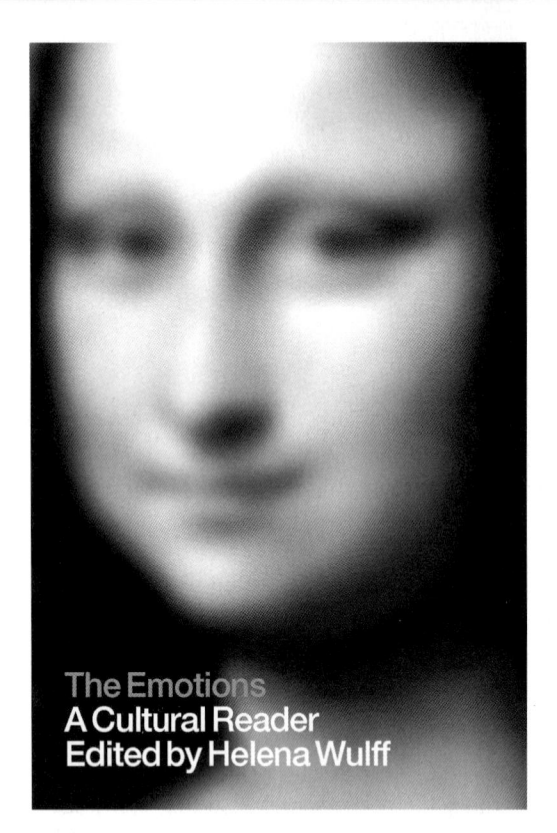

Edited by Helena Wulff

Emotions are a loaded topic. From love and hate to grief, fear and envy, emotions are increasingly understood as driving forces in social life. *The Emotions: A Cultural Reader* applies a cross-cultural perspective on emotions. It examines the fact that emotions are socially and culturally constructed, while highlighting problems of comparison and translation of local terms and emotional experiences.

Are emotions cultural or universal? To what extent are there culturally distinct emotions? *The Emotions* closes the traditional Western gap where emotions are separated from rationality and thought: the heart versus mind debate. By presenting both classic essays and new cutting-edge chapters from anthropology, sociology and psychology with important contributions from philosophy and neuroscience, the volume connects a rich range of cross-cultural studies to form a thriving interdisciplinary debate on emotions.

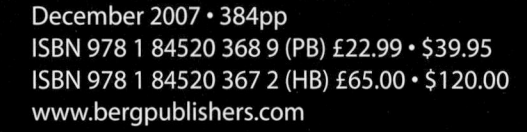

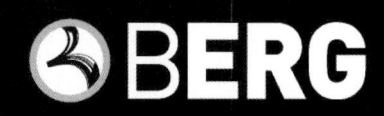

December 2007 • 384pp
ISBN 978 1 84520 368 9 (PB) £22.99 • $39.95
ISBN 978 1 84520 367 2 (HB) £65.00 • $120.00
www.bergpublishers.com

BERG

Luigi Russolo's Art of Noises

Estorick Collection of Modern Italian Art, London, October 4–December 17, 2006

James Mansell

James Mansell is a Postgraduate Fellow at the University of Manchester. He is currently preparing a doctoral thesis on the modernist experience of sound in London and Paris, 1880–1940.
James.Mansell@manchester.ac.uk

The perceptual shock of life in the early twentieth century's great cities has been understood in overwhelmingly visual terms. From the blasé glance of Georg Simmel's street-walker to the god-like elevation of Michel de Certeau's city-planner, few have disagreed with Walter Benjamin's assertion that "interpersonal relationships in big cities are distinguished by a marked preponderance of the activity of the eye over the activity of the ear" (1997: 38). Yet we find a contemporary of Benjamin's inviting us to "walk together through a great modern capital, with the ear more attentive than the eye" (Russolo 1986: 26). This Italian Futurist also invites us to "vary the pleasures of our sensibilities by distinguishing among the gurglings of water, air and gas inside metallic pipes," and "the rumbling and rattlings of engines breathing with obvious animal spirits" (Russolo 1986: 26).

Luigi Russolo (1885–1947) shared with other Futurists an interest in the urban and the technological, and a desire to create an art movement which harnessed the totality

Exhibition Reviews

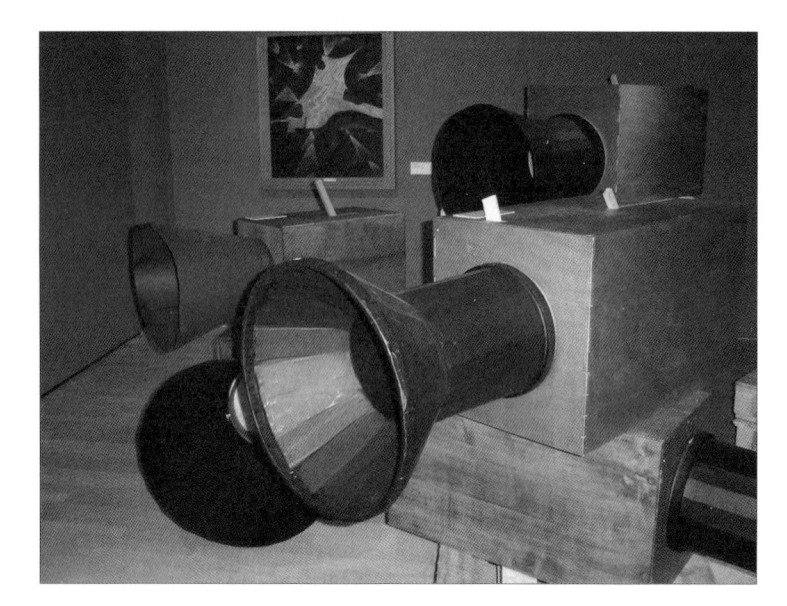

Figure 1
Reconstructed *intonarumori*, installation view. Photograph courtesy Estorick Collection, London.

of modernity's sensations. He is remembered principally for the pioneering book in which the above suggestions are made, *The Art of Noises*, published in 1916. To accompany this manifesto, Russolo famously built "noise intoners" (*intonarumori*), which acoustically reproduced urban sounds and included among their number "the howler," "the buzzer" and "the whistler," the latter of which, for example, produced a sound "similar to the humming of electric motors" (Lombardi 2006a: 119). These "proto-electronic experiences," as Daniele Lombardi describes them, "tended toward the construction of refined instruments intended to enrich the symphonic timbre of the orchestra" (2006b: 111), with the intoners being combined with conventional instruments in a number of Futurist concerts, including one in London, in the years immediately after World War I. In using everyday city sounds as the raw materials of musical composition, Russolo had anticipated the electro-acoustic music movement begun in the studios of *musique concrète* in the 1940s.

Less familiar, though, is Russolo's work as a painter. In fact, as the Estorick Collection's exhibition demonstrates, his work in the visual and aural arts was interdependent and mutually constitutive. The exhibition was remarkable for presenting Russolo's major paintings together for the first time alongside replicas of the noise intoners, which were demonstrated to visitors by gallery staff. So, with the peculiar aural backdrop produced by a "crackler" or a "croaker," one is left to consider Russolo's 1911 painting *Music*, which seems to hold the key to understanding the role of sound in his aesthetic theory. Foregrounded is a figure resembling Beethoven hunched at a piano, whose music is represented by a curving blue stream which snakes across the center of the canvas. The background includes

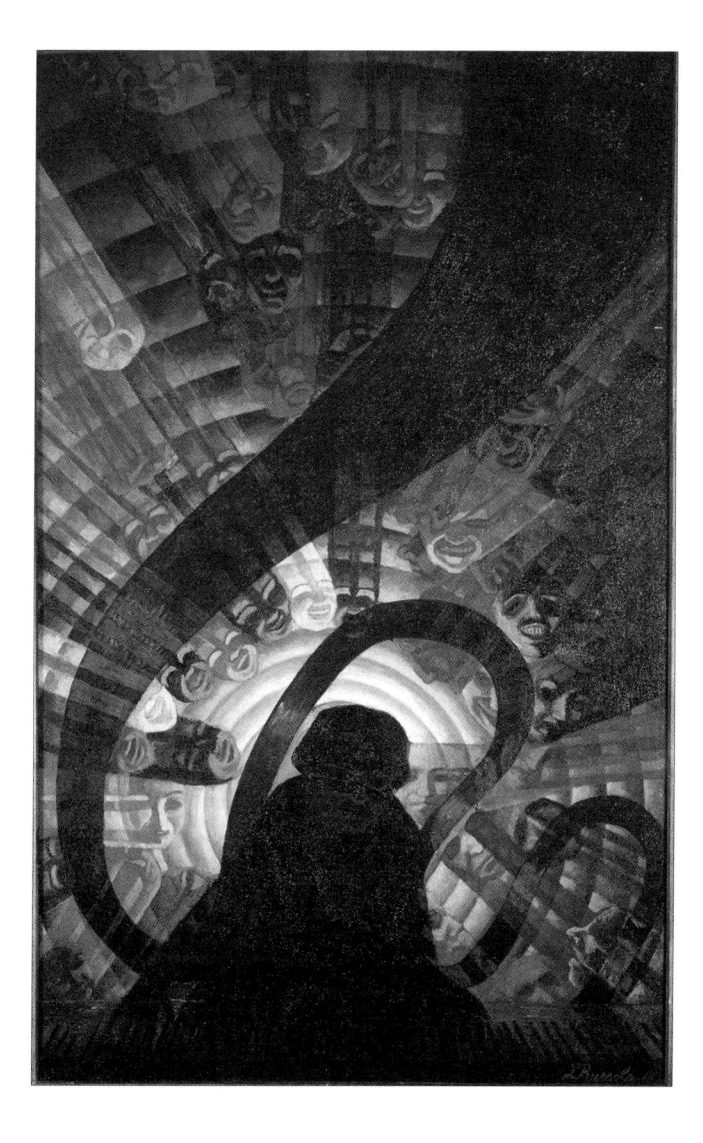

Figure 2
Luigi Russolo, *Music*, 1911. Oil on canvas, 225 x 140 cm. Collection of Estorick Collection. Photograph courtesy Estorick Collection, London.

concentric circles representing vibrating sound waves and masks whose trails of red, green or yellow seem to stand for the multiple emotional states of the music (Tagliapietra 2006: 26–7).

The painting contains two important clues to Russolo's aesthetic inspiration. The first is the esoteric spirituality of the work, which as the exhibition demonstrates, became an increasingly important interest for Russolo in the later phases of his creative life. For example, Rudolph Steiner's 1922 book *Theosophy: An Introduction to the Supersensible Knowledge of the World and the Destination of Man* is placed in the exhibition in acknowledgment of its influence on Russolo's own *Al di làdella materia* ("Beyond Matter") (1938). Steiner's esoteric theory of color is useful in understanding the use of color in *Music*. He explains that "exactly as processes in space can be seen with the sensible eye as color-phenomena, so can ... soul and spiritual processes become, by means of the inner senses, perceptions which are analogous to the sensible color-phenomena" (Steiner 1970: 119). Blue shades, as in *Music*, "appear in intensely devotional moods of soul. The more a man places his Self in the service of a cause," continues Steiner, "the more pronounced become the blue shades" (1970: 123).

Lombardi identifies Russolo's "spiritualist course" as one which "considered form with a sensibility close to that of the abstractionists and Constructivists in the sphere of painting, in the name of a synaesthesia that found its own figuration in analogies between visual and auditory impulses" (2006b: 111). Esoteric spiritualities such as theosophy, revived at the end of the nineteenth century (Owen 2004), are an under-researched aspect of modernism's intellectual foundation, and are an example of a trajectory in which visual and aural phenomena were considered to be bound together as interdependent aspects of psychic life.

The second clue which *Music* holds is the influence of the French philosopher Henri Bergson. Marianne Martin suggests that the painting comes "close to illustrating Bergson's conception of 'psychic duration' as memory which links the past with the present and future" (1968: 89). Bergson's pure duration (*durée*) privileges lived experience over the spatial abstractions of modern time as projected on the clock face. Bergson's theory that "both the past and the present states" should be formed "into an organic whole" (2001: 100) is echoed in a Futurist exhibition note of 1912, of which Russolo was co-author:

> This [simultaneity of states of mind] implies the simultaneousness of the ambient and, therefore, the dislocation and dismemberment of objects, the scattering and fusion of details, freed from accepted logic, and independent from one another. In order to make the spectator live in the center of the picture ... the picture must be the synthesis of *what one remembers* and of *what one sees* (Tagliapietra 2006: 31, emphasis in original).

Bergson considered music to be the art which best expresses memory and pure duration, which he likens to "the notes of a tune, melting, so to speak, into one another" (2001: 100). Russolo describes *Music*'s blue swathe in strongly Bergsonian terms: "the unravelling of the melodic line in time is translated into that deep blue beam, which, snaking through space, dominates and envelops the entire painting" (Tagliapietra 2006: 27). This insight into the close connection between sound, memory and perceptual experience, as evidenced in many Futurist paintings, was formative to Russolo's approach in his art of noises. Seeing Russolo's paintings alongside his noise experiments recreates at least some of the synaesthetic impressions which are at the heart of his urban landscapes and soundscapes. The exhibition was a unique opportunity to consider not only the unity of visual and aural expressivity in Russolo's work but also an alternative history of modernism and modern perception that incorporates auditory culture as a crucial element in the experience and representation of urban modernity.

References

Benjamin, Walter. 1997. *Charles Baudelaire: A Lyric Poet in the Era of High Capitalism*. Translated by Harry Zohn. London: Verso.

Bergson, Henri. 2001. *Time and Free Will: An Essay on the Immediate Data of Consciousness*. Translated by F. L. Pogson. New York: Dover Publications.

Lombardi, Daniele. 2006a. "Description of the *Intonarumori* in a Letter from Russolo to Pratella." In Anna Gasparato and Franco Tagliapietra (eds), *Luigi Russolo: Life and Works of a Futurist*. Translated by Chiara Acanfora, et al. Milan: Skiara.

——— 2006b. "So Much Noise for Nothing?" In Anna Gasparato and Franco Tagliapietra (eds), *Luigi Russolo: Life and Works of a Futurist*. Translated by Chiara Acanfora, et al. Milan: Skiara.

Martin, Marianne W. 1968. *Futurist Art and Theory 1909-1915*. Oxford: Clarendon Press.

Owen, Alex. 2004. *The Place of Enchantment: British Occultism and the Culture of the Modern*. Chicago: Chicago University Press.

Russolo, Luigi. 1938. *Al di là della materia : alla ricerca del vero; alla ricerca del bello; alla ricerca del bene*. Milan: Fratelli Bocca.

——— 1986. *The Art of Noises*. Translated by Barclay Brown. New York: Pendragon Press.

Steiner, Rudolph. 1970. *Theosophy: An Introduction to the Supersensible Knowledge of the World and the Destination of Man*. London: Rudolph Steiner Press.

Tagliapietra, Franco. 2006. "From Symbolist Influences to Futurist Art and Theory: Etchings and Paintings." In Anna Gasparato and Franco Tagliapietra (eds), *Luigi Russolo: Life and Works of a Futurist*. Translated by Chiara Acanfora, et al. Milan: Skiara.

The Design of Everyday Life

Elizabeth Shove, Matthew Watson, Jack Ingram and Martin Hand

192pp • 234 x 156 mm
PB 978 1 84520 683 3 **£19.99 • $34.95**
HB 978 1 84520 682 6 **£55.00 • $99.95**

"This book uses the everyday artefact to break new intellectual ground for consumption studies, design analysis, and the field of material culture. Based in close empirical observation of social practice, it helps bring a new sociology of the artefact into being. It is creative, fresh, and original."—HARVEY MOLOTCH, New York University

How do common household items such as basic plastic house wares or high-tech digital cameras transform our daily lives? *The Design of Everyday Life* considers this question in detail, from the design of products through to their use in the home.

Drawing on interviews with consumers themselves, the authors look at how everyday objects, ranging from screwdrivers to photo management software, are used on a practical level. Closely investigating the design, production and use of mass-market goods, the authors offer new interpretations of how consumers' needs are met and manufactured. They examine the dynamic interaction of products with everyday practices.

The Design of Everyday Life presents a pathbreaking analysis of the sociology of objects, illuminating the connections between design and consumption.

BERG

Between Art and Science

Patrizia Di Bello

Making Sense of Art, Making Art of Sense Conference. Organized by Francesca Bacci, Department of Art and Centre for Visual Studies, Oxford University, and David Melcher, Department of Psychology, Oxford Brookes University. October 27–9, 2006, Science Oxford, Oxford, UK

Patrizia Di Bello is a lecturer in the School of History of Art, Film and Visual Media, Birkbeck, University of London. She is author of *Women's Albums and Photography in Victorian Britain: Ladies, Mothers and Flirts* (Ashgate), and is editing a collection on *Other Than The Visual: Art, History and the Senses*.
p.dibello@bbk.ac.uk

We remember conferences for the papers we heard, the people we met, perhaps the interesting locations. My enduring memories of *Making Sense of Art, Making Art of Sense* are associated with smell: the strange scent of Oswaldo Marcia's *Smellscape* installation drifting from the exhibition next door, and Professor Tim Jacob sniffing his armpit, like a teenager on a date worried about BO, to demonstrate how to "reset" one's sense of smell once it has become habituated to a particular odor.

This was a truly interdisciplinary and multisensorial event, where academic papers interacted with art works, synesthetic performances, taste and sound demonstrations (crisps taste better when their crunchy sound is amplified

– now we know why children insist on eating them with their mouth open) and a multicolored conference dinner – which I had to miss, but heard much about, especially the blue soup. You could practically smell the intellectual excitement, the feeling we were contributing to a "sensory revolution" – a paradigm shift in ways of thinking about culture, the body and the important role of *all* of the senses in shaping both.

The conference brought together scientists, art historians, curators and artists working on the role of the senses in the creation and reception of art. Its very structure questioned hierarchies between the senses and between the disciplines that construct them as separate. The sessions were organized around touch, audition, smell and taste, synesthesia and vision – each being addressed by a scientist and a humanities scholar. This juxtaposition generated much productive dialogue between the papers and within the audience. Explicitly or implicitly many of the papers questioned how and why vision and audition have been privileged in Western cultures as the senses that can be addressed through specialized, monosensorial discourses such as "pure music" or "the visual arts." Here, I want to comment on some of the common themes: the plasticity of the senses in their interaction with culture; their inherent cross- and multi-modality; and the value of studying the senses through a synthesis of as yet separate disciplines.

The scientists seemed to agree that the senses are shaped by environmental, cultural and social circumstances rather than being solely innate. They need to be, as they need to adapt to changing circumstances to work efficiently as tools of survival. The extent of their plasticity, however, was much debated. Do our senses passively register the world, or do they make it for us, by shaping our perceptions? How do cultural and gender differences impact on neurological research? Is women's better sense of smell, for example, a question of nature or nurture? Is it valid to generalize in the absence of truly multicultural research? The challenge for neuropsychology is to construct non-Western models for the study of the senses. But can commercially funded research meet this challenge? If, for example, the study of touch is related to designing more purchase-enticing packaging, as Charles Spence's paper indicated, the tactility of cultures not yet co-opted into Western consumerism is irrelevant. More widely, how can we study the senses, if the senses of those who study them are as culturally constructed as those under scrutiny? From my perspective as an art historian, this poses exciting if difficult research questions: if our present sensual perception of music, paintings, sculptures – or any surviving material culture – cannot be assumed to be the same as that of the past, how can we reconstruct not only a "period eye" – Michael Baxandall's term (1972) – but a whole "period" sensorium? What seems clear is the value of bringing together science and the humanities to tackle these issues.

If the senses are plastic, subject to change and determined by previous experiences, so are their pleasures. David Melcher's paper gave further scientific support to the idea that visual perception is not a passive optical mirror of nature but an interactive, multisensory and embodied activity. Acts of imagination are crucial in creating what we perceive as continuous vision scenes, by making up, for example, for "blind spots" – split seconds in the scanning process in which we do not actually see anything. Memory plays an important role, relating vision as it happens to previous images, in order to register difference or recognition. As recognition is neurologically pleasurable, what we find attractive is related to what we have been looking at before – to our "diet" of visual images. The notion that we are not only what we eat but also what we see has considerable implications for the ongoing debates on the effects of images recurring in the media, whether of violence, exploitative sex, or emaciated bodies. It does not account, however, for how we find pleasure also in dissonance and surprise. Perhaps these are needed to exercise the flexibility of our senses to keep them adaptable and responsive to change. Activities separated out from the everyday and elevated to the category of art might provide a safe, self-contained context in which to experience sensual dissonance and surprise as pleasurable.

The other thread running through the whole of the conference was that of the interconnectedness of the senses. Visual stimuli, for example, activate parts of the brain associated with processing other sense data – seeing movement in a picture activates parts of the brain that process motion, while touching activates visual recognition areas, even in the blind. Equally, all cultural apparatus organizing and enabling sensorial experience is multisensory – as Simon Shaw-Miller's paper highlighted, music is always also visual, tactile and embodied; it can be felt by deaf people. More generally, the look and feel of musical instruments and media, from drums to the iPod, is of crucial importance in the development of music – audition organized as a cultural practice.

The senses have been separated, ranked and studied, by producing disciplined bodies as both subjects and objects of investigation. Yet sensations – the actions and productions of the senses – are synesthetic. They work both in isolation and together, multi-, trans- and intersensorially. As the result of interactions between nature and culture, between body and mind, the senses are where these distinctions become problematic, blurred and impossible to maintain. Yet splitting the senses seems to be important to create disciplines and to establish notions of disciplined behavior – at art exhibitions, concerts, at the table, or in the laboratory and the lecture room. Splitting the senses, at least in Western cultures, seems to be fundamental in defining a "clean and proper" self or identity, at both conscious and unconscious levels.

As David Howes argued, neurosystems are created by material cultures; any aesthetic and any science of the senses must be multi- and cross modal, as their integration is shaped by cultural practices as well as neural processes. If the plasticity of the senses is cross modal, we should start with the notion of synesthesia not as a neurological exception but as the basic modus operandi of all perceptions before moving on to study individual senses. An understanding of the cultural organization of the senses should precede psychological or neurological investigation.

This conference was an important attempt to move forward from a cross- or multidisciplinary approach – as Shaw-Miller described it, this is an unstable, often tense relation between disciplines that remain separate even when they move politely in the same direction – towards a synthesis where disciplines merge to become one. Such a synthesis, however, might cause some resistance and an anxiety associated with loss of control: the scientist, like the art connoisseur, needs a demarcated field to establish mastery, as argued by Fiona Candlin in her paper on "Touch and the Separation of the Senses."

This event successfully generated an interdisciplinary platform where science and the humanities can develop in dialogue and create a new, interdisciplinary sensory field of investigation. It also highlighted the enormous potential of an understanding of cultures based on how they interact with and affect us through our senses. We might not all have the historical or theoretical confidence to feel we understand art, but we are all equipped with a very sophisticated sensorium we can use as a laboratory. The importance of sensual exploration and experimentation for its own sake is recognized in children's toys and education, but in Western cultures is too often forgotten in adult life, reduced to shopping for novelty.

The conference left us all buzzing with ideas and wanting to discuss them some more – so that writing this is a particular pleasure. A book based on the conference is going to be published by Oxford University Press, edited by its organizers, art historian Francesca Bacci and psychologist David Melcher, under the title of *Art and the Senses*. All told, this was a very productive as well as enjoyable event.

References

Baxandall, Michael. 1972. *Painting and Experience in Fifteenth Century Italy*. Oxford: Clarendon Press.